Stroke - Management Pearls

Edited by Amit Agrawal

Published in London, United Kingdom

Stroke - Management Pearls
http://dx.doi.org/10.5772/intechopen.108084
Edited by Amit Agrawal

Contributors
Takayuki Kodama, Ken Kitai, Aleksandr Urakov, Varvara Sokolova, Aleksandr Samorodov, Adeolu Morawo, Andrés J. Ursa Herguedas, María Pellón Olmedo, Dragos Catalin Jianu, Silviana Nina Jianu, Nicoleta Iacob, Traian Flavius Dan, Georgiana Munteanu, Anca Elena Gogu, Ligia Petrica, Yukari Hisaka, Allan Paulo Blaquera, Kensaku Takase, Tetsuya Tanioka, Þórður Helgason, Kristjana Ósk Kristinsdóttir, Samuel Ruipérez-Campillo, Amit Agrawal, Luis Rafael Moscote-Salazar, Md. Moshiur Rahman

First published in London, United Kingdom, 2023 by IntechOpen
IntechOpen is the global imprint of INTECHOPEN LIMITED, registered in England and Wales, registration number: 11086078, 5 Princes Gate Court, London, SW7 2QJ, United Kingdom

British Library Cataloguing-in-Publication Data
A catalogue record for this book is available from the British Library

Additional hard and PDF copies can be obtained from orders@intechopen.com

Stroke - Management Pearls
Edited by Amit Agrawal
p. cm.
Print ISBN 978-1-80356-786-0
Online ISBN 978-1-80356-787-7
eBook (PDF) ISBN 978-1-80356-842-3

For EU product safety concerns:
IN TECH d.o.o., Prolaz Marije Krucifikse Kozulić 3, 51000 Rijeka, Croatia,
info@intechopen.com or visit our website at intechopen.com.

Meet the editor

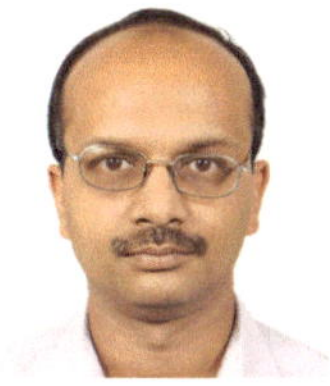

Dr. Amit Agrawal completed his neurosurgery training at the National Institute of Mental Health and Neurosciences, Bangalore, India, in 2003. He is a self-motivated, enthusiastic, and results-oriented professional with more than 18 years of rich experience in research and development as well as teaching and mentoring in the field of neurosurgery. He is proficient in managing and leading teams to run successful process operations and has experience in developing procedures and service standards of excellence. Dr. Agrawal has attended and participated in many international and national symposiums and conferences and delivered lectures on vivid topics. He has published more than 750 articles in national and international journals. His expertise is in identifying training needs, designing training modules, and executing the same while working with limited resources. He has excellent communication, presentation, and interpersonal skills with proven abilities in teaching and training for various academic and professional courses. Presently, Dr. Agrawal is working at the All-India Institute of Medical Sciences, Bhopal, Madhya Pradesh, India.

Contents

Preface IX

Chapter 1 1
Introductory Chapter: Neurosurgical Management of Intracerebral Hemorrhage
by Luis Rafael Moscote-Salazar, Md. Moshiur Rahman and Amit Agrawal

Chapter 2 9
Perspective Chapter: Clinical Standard of a Geriatric Patient as a Virtual Target for Correction of Pharmacotherapy of Hypertension and Stroke in the Elderly
by Aleksandr Urakov, Aleksandr Samorodov and Varvara Sokolova

Chapter 3 25
Clinical Usefulness of Real-time Sensory Compensation Feedback Training on Sensorimotor Dysfunction after Stroke
by Takayuki Kodama and Ken Kitai

Chapter 4 51
Intravenous Thrombolysis in Acute Ischemic Stroke
by Adeolu Morawo

Chapter 5 65
Cerebral Veins and Dural Sinuses Thrombosis: State-of-the-Art Diagnosis
by Dragos Catalin Jianu, Silviana Nina Jianu, Nicoleta Iacob, Traian Flavius Dan, Georgiana Munteanu, Anca Elena Gogu and Ligia Petrica

Chapter 6 99
Action on the Cerebral Vascular Endothelium in the Prevention of Stroke
by Andrés J. Ursa Herguedas and María Pellón Olmedo

Chapter 7 115
Key Points of Nursing Care for Patients with Acute Stroke
by Yukari Hisaka, Allan Paulo Blaquera, Kensaku Takase and Tetsuya Tanioka

Chapter 8 131
Quantifying Spasticity: A Review
by Kristjana Ósk Kristinsdóttir, Samuel Ruipérez-Campillo and Þórður Helgason

Preface

Stroke is among the leading causes of morbidity and mortality globally and its incidence is on the rise. It is increasingly recognized that an understanding of various clinical presentations among clinicians and other stakeholders is extremely important to achieve better outcomes in stroke patients. Apart from the obvious clinical deficits, the subtle signs and clinical symptoms of stroke, including acute dizziness and vertigo, may provide a clue about ischemic events involving the brain. Because of the subtlety of stroke's clinical presentation, it is challenging to diagnose in clinics as well as in emergency departments. This book provides a practical approach and a summary of recommendations for the management of stroke patients. A detailed history and clinical examinations are the mainstays of stroke diagnosis followed by a CT scan, which is the initial investigation of choice in most settings. CT can be followed by MRI, particularly diffusion-weighted (DWI) sequences and other investigations, to assess the cerebral cranial vasculature and formulate a management strategy. Overall, the diagnosis and management of stroke require multimodal strategies and a multidisciplinary approach to make the diagnosis and deliver optimal treatment, which will include medical as well as surgical management in select cases. The book helps to understand and explore current advances, including the identification of the molecular characteristics that determine the malignant phenotype that may further help to develop effective management strategies, including immunotherapy. There is a scope for future research where global leaders can come together to develop affordable, sustainable, and uniformly available options to prevent as well as manage stroke.

Amit Agrawal
Department of Neurosurgery,
All India Institute of Medical Sciences,
Bhopal, India

Chapter 1

Introductory Chapter: Neurosurgical Management of Intracerebral Hemorrhage

Luis Rafael Moscote-Salazar, Md. Moshiur Rahman and Amit Agrawal

1. Introduction

Primary spontaneous intracerebral haemorrhage (SICH) can lead to fatal outcomes and in survivors can be cause of significant morbidity and long-term disability [1]. In up to 90% patient's arterial hypertension or amyloid angiopathy gas been attributed as the cause of bleeding [2]. Important points to differentiate primary SICH from secondary SICH include primary SICH usually involve basal ganglia, thalamus in patients with history of hypertension [2–5]. The increase in life expectancy and increase in aging population it can be anticipated the burden of SICH shall continue to increase [6, 7] with an increase in overall lifetime cost for management of these patients [8]. The role of neurosurgical intervention and available options in the management of spontaneous SICH is not only increasing but also able to improve overall outcomes. We exclude the discussion for the management of spontaneous cerebellar hematomas as these are special subtypes have relative better clinical outcome [2].

2. Clinical characteristics

Each patient needs to evaluated in details including details clinical history and clinical examination particularly neurological deficits and extent of the deficits [2]. Clinical characteristics of the SICH depends on the size, location of the bleed presence or absence of hydrocephalus. General manifestations include sign of raised intracranial pressure i.e., headache, vomiting, seizures, and altered levels of consciousness (including coma in severe cases) [2]. The two common risk factors for SICH include systemic arterial hypertension and cerebral amyloid angiopathy [9, 10].

3. Diagnosis

Primary SICH needs to be differentiated from other causes of haemorrhages i.e., from secondary SICH (for example traumatic ICH, tumours with haemorrhage, vascular malformations, and pharmacological causes of SICH) [2]. Whenever a SICH is suspected, CT scan brain will provide the details regarding presence of blood including its location with sensitivity of more than 95%, in some patients [11, 12] CT scan may not show the blood, in these cases MR can help in finding the blood particularly with T2* and proton weighted sequences [12, 13]. In cases where a secondary cause of intracerebral haemorrhage is suspected CT and MR can be supplemented with MR-angiography, CT-angiography, or if necessary conventional digital subtraction angiography [11].

4. Management

Management may range from medical management and observation alone to aggressive surgical intervention that may include evacuation of the hematoma and/or decompressive craniectomy [14–26]. Standard conservative management and management of patient who is a candidate for surgery include stabilization of airway, breathing, circulation stabilization, control of blood pressure followed by measures to reduce intracranial pressure either anti-oedema measures or surgical evacuation of the hematoma and prevention of secondary complications (pneumonia, DVT, urinary tract infection, pressure ulcers) [27]. For example, surgery may not be advisable in patients with large thalamic haemorrhages or haemorrhages extending into the brain stem in a patient who has poor neurological grade [2].

5. Surgical management

In addition to medical management options, a range of several invasive neurosurgical approaches have been described for clot removal and to reduce mass effect. These approached include open craniotomy to evacuate hematoma with or without decompressive craniectomy, image-guided stereotactic endoscopic aspiration, minimally invasive methods for thrombolysis and placement of external ventricular drainage (in cases of intraventricular extension of the clot of associated hydrocephalus) have been described [27]. Decision to perform surgery can be influenced by the facilities available, expertise and patient related factors, the surgical options include open craniotomy and evacuation of the hematoma, endoscopic evacuation of the hematoma, stereotactic evacuation of the hematoma, CSF diversion procedures like EVD of VP shunt if there in extension into the ventricles or associated obstructive hydrocephalus.

6. Scope of neurosurgical intervention

The role of neurosurgical interventions has been expanding in the management of SICH however there are many challenges ahead and many questions needs to be answered. For example, any follow up intervention cannot reverse the primary injury [27] but at the same time it can help to minimize secondary injury. Evacuating the hematoma can be a lifesaving procedure, however there is a need to further understand how can we improve the overall quality of life of the survivors. The decision to perform surgical evacuation can be weighed in a case-to-case basis. For examples Reichart [2].

- Small haemorrhages involving basal ganglia with minimal or absent neurological deficits can be managed conservatively

- In large hematomas where a whole hemisphere is involved, patient is an elderly with poor neurological grade, surgery may be lifesaving but prognosis remains poor hence surgery may not be advisable

- Conscious patients with hematomas between 30 and 50 ml, deep location and without mass effect can be managed conservatively. However, if secondary neurological deterioration occurs and the volume of hematoma increases and size may be of 50–60 ml, open craniotomy and evacuating of the hematoma can be considered

- Young patients with a moderate or large lobar haemorrhage who are clinically deteriorating may need surgical intervention

- SICH associated with a structural lesion such as an aneurysm, arteriovenous malformation or cavernous angioma may need surgical intervention.

7. Challenges

Although recent advancements both in terms of medical and surgical management of these patients have resulted in improved survivals however overall functional outcomes remains compromised [27–34]. Many studies have explored the role of surgery in the management of spontaneous intracerebral hematomas [35]. However, the generalization of the results and management of individual patients remains both controversial and challenging.

8. Conclusions

There is a need for evidence-based algorithms which can better address management options as well as overall functional outcomes of these patients, where the individual patient regain functional independence as well as can be integrated into the society. As investigators, in addition to the development of post event management protocols and factors facilitating the neuronal recovery, but also to focus on techniques those can detect high risk patients to develop SICH and strategies like risk factor modifications to prevent episodes of SICH which can potentially be fatal or can leave the patients with severe disability.

Author details

Luis Rafael Moscote-Salazar[1], Md. Moshiur Rahman[2] and Amit Agrawal[3*]

1 Colombian Clinical Research Group in Neurocritical Care, Bogota, Colombia

2 Department of Neurosurgery, Holy Family Red Crescent Medical College Hospital, Dhaka, Bangladesh

3 Department of Neurosurgery, All India Institute of Medical Sciences, Bhopal, Madhya Pradesh, India

*Address all correspondence to: dramitagrawal@gmail.com; dramitagrawal@hotmail.com

References

[1] Katan M, Luft A. Global burden of stroke. Seminars in Neurology. 2018;**38**(2):208-211. DOI: 10.1055/s-0038-1649503

[2] Reichart R, Frank S. Intracerebral hemorrhage, indication for surgical treatment and surgical techniques. The Open Critical Care Medicine Journal. 2011;**4**(1):68-71

[3] Naidech AM. Intracranial hemorrhage.American Journal of Respiratory and Critical Care Medicine. 1 Nov 2011;**184**(9):998-1006. DOI: 10.1164/rccm.201103-0475CI. PMID: 22167847; PMCID: PMC3361326

[4] Masuda J, Tanaka K, Ueda K, Omae T. Autopsy study of incidence and distribution of cerebral amyloid angiopathy in Hisayama, Japan. Stroke. 1988;**19**(2):205-210. DOI: 10.1161/01.str.19.2.205

[5] Elijovich L, Patel PV, Hemphill JC. Intracerebral hemorrhage. Seminars in Neurology. 2008;**28**(5):657-667. DOI: 10.1055/s-0028-1105974

[6] Feigin VL, Krishnamurthi RV, Parmar P, et al. Update on the Global Burden of Ischemic and Hemorrhagic Stroke in 1990-2013: The GBD 2013 Study. Neuroepidemiology. 2015;**45**(3):161-176. DOI: 10.1159/000441085

[7] Feigin VL, Lawes CMM, Bennett DA, Anderson CS. Stroke epidemiology: A review of population-based studies of incidence, prevalence, and case-fatality in the late 20th century. Lancet Neurology. 2003;**2**(1):43-53. DOI: 10.1016/s1474-4422(03)00266-7

[8] Cha Y-J. The economic burden of stroke based on South Korea's National Health Insurance Claims Database. Intenational Journal of Health Policy Management. 2018;7(10):904-909. DOI: 10.15171/ijhpm.2018.42

[9] Ariesen MJ, Claus SP, Rinkel GJE, Algra A. Risk factors for intracerebral hemorrhage in the general population: A systematic review. Stroke. 2003;**34**(8):2060-2065. DOI: 10.1161/01.STR.0000080678.09344.8D

[10] Yamada M. Cerebral amyloid angiopathy: Emerging concepts. Journal of Stroke. 2015;**17**(1):17-30. DOI: 10.5853/jos.2015.17.1.17

[11] van Straaten ECW, Scheltens P, Barkhof F. MRI and CT in the diagnosis of vascular dementia. Journal of the Neurological Sciences. 2004;**226**(1-2):9-12. DOI: 10.1016/j.jns.2004.09.003

[12] Fiebach JB, Schellinger PD, Gass A, et al. Stroke magnetic resonance imaging is accurate in hyperacute intracerebral hemorrhage: A multicenter study on the validity of stroke imaging. Stroke. 2004;**35**(2):502-506. DOI: 10.1161/01.STR.0000114203.75678.88

[13] Kidwell CS, Chalela JA, Saver JL, et al. Comparison of MRI and CT for detection of acute intracerebral hemorrhage. Journal of the American Medical Association. 2004;**292**(15):1823-1830. DOI: 10.1001/jama.292.15.1823

[14] Raafat M, Ragab OA, Abdelwahab OM, Salama MM, Hafez MA. Early versus delayed surgical evacuation of spontaneous supratentorial intracerebral hematoma: A prospective cohort study. Surgical Neurological International. 2020;**11**:145. DOI: 10.25259/SNI_103_2020

[15] Schirmer CM, Hoit DA, Malek AM. Decompressive hemicraniectomy for

the treatment of intractable intracranial hypertension after aneurysmal subarachnoid hemorrhage. Stroke. 2007;**38**(3):987-992. DOI: 10.1161/01.STR.0000257962.58269.e2

[16] Wong GKC, Boet R, Ng SCP, et al. Ultra-early (within 24 hours) aneurysm treatment after subarachnoid hemorrhage. World Neurosurgery. 2012;**77**(2):311-315. DOI: 10.1016/j.wneu.2011.09.025

[17] X-q Z, Z-m Z, X-l Y, Zhang K, Cai H, Ling F. Exploring the optimal operation time for patients with hypertensive intracerebral hemorrhage: Tracking the expression and progress of cell apoptosis of prehematomal brain tissues. Chinese Medical Journal. 2010;**123**(10):1246-1250

[18] Auer LM, Holzer P, Ascher PW, Heppner F. Endoscopic neurosurgery. Acta Neurochirurgica. 1988;**90**(1-2):1-14. DOI: 10.1007/BF01541260

[19] Cho D-Y, Chen C-C, Chang C-S, Lee W-Y, Tso M. Endoscopic surgery for spontaneous basal ganglia hemorrhage: Comparing endoscopic surgery, stereotactic aspiration, and craniotomy in noncomatose patients. Surgical Neurology. 2006;**65**(6):547-555; discussion 555-556. DOI: 10.1016/j.surneu.2005.09.032

[20] Nishihara T, Morita A, Teraoka A, Kirino T. Endoscopy-guided removal of spontaneous intracerebral hemorrhage: Comparison with computer tomography-guided stereotactic evacuation. Child's Nervous System. 2007;**23**(6):677-683. DOI: 10.1007/s00381-007-0325-6

[21] Matsumoto K, Hondo H. CT-guided stereotaxic evacuation of hypertensive intracerebral hematomas. Journal of Neurosurgery. 1984;**61**(3):440-448. DOI: 10.3171/jns.1984.61.3.0440

[22] Murthy JMK, Chowdary GVS, Murthy TVRK, Bhasha PSA, Naryanan TJ. Decompressive craniectomy with clot evacuation in large hemispheric hypertensive intracerebral hemorrhage. Neurocritical Care. 2005;**2**(3):258-262. DOI: 10.1385/ncc:2:3:258

[23] Teernstra OPM, Evers SMA, Lodder J, et al. Stereotactic treatment of intracerebral hematoma by means of a plasminogen activator: A multicenter randomized controlled trial (SICHPA). Stroke. 2003;**34**(4):968-974. DOI: 10.1161/01.STR.0000063367.52044.40

[24] Kim IS, Son BC, Lee SW, Sung JH, Hong JT. Comparison of frame-based and frameless stereotactic hematoma puncture and subsequent fibrinolytic therapy for the treatment of supratentorial deep seated spontaneous intracerebral hemorrhage. Minimally Invasive Neurosurgery. 2007;**50**(2):86-90. DOI: 10.1055/s-2007-982503

[25] Thiex R, Rohde V, Rohde I, et al. Frame-based and frameless stereotactic hematoma puncture and subsequent fibrinolytic therapy for the treatment of spontaneous intracerebral hemorrhage. Journal of Neurology. 2004;**251**(12):1443-1450. DOI: 10.1007/s00415-004-0554-5

[26] Sumer MM, Açikgöz B, Akpinar G. External ventricular drainage for acute obstructive hydrocephalus developing following spontaneous intracerebral haemorrhages. Neurological Sciences. 2002;**23**(1):29-33. DOI: 10.1007/s100720200020

[27] de Oliveira Manoel AL. Surgery for spontaneous intracerebral hemorrhage. Critical care (London, England). 2020;**24**(1):45. DOI: 10.1186/s13054-020-2749-2

[28] Linares G, Mayer SA. Hypothermia for the treatment of ischemic and

hemorrhagic stroke. Critical Care Medicine. 2009;**37**(7 Suppl):S243-S249. DOI: 10.1097/CCM.0b013e3181aa5de1

[29] Anderson CS, Heeley E, Huang Y, et al. Rapid blood-pressure lowering in patients with acute intracerebral hemorrhage. The New England Journal of Medicine. 2013;**368**(25):2355-2365. DOI: 10.1056/NEJMoa1214609

[30] Qureshi AI, Palesch YY, Barsan WG, et al. Intensive blood-pressure lowering in patients with acute cerebral hemorrhage. The New England Journal of Medicine. 2016;**375**(11):1033-1043. DOI: 10.1056/NEJMoa1603460

[31] Mayer SA, Brun NC, Begtrup K, et al. Efficacy and safety of recombinant activated factor VII for acute intracerebral hemorrhage. The New England Journal of Medicine. 2008;**358**(20):2127-2137. DOI: 10.1056/NEJMoa0707534

[32] Sprigg N, Flaherty K, Appleton JP, et al. Tranexamic acid for hyperacute primary IntraCerebral Haemorrhage (TICH-2): An international randomised, placebo-controlled, phase 3 superiority trial. Lancet. 2018;**391**(10135):2107-2115. DOI: 10.1016/S0140-6736(18)31033-X

[33] Wong JM, Ziewacz JE, Ho AL, et al. Patterns in neurosurgical adverse events: Open cerebrovascular neurosurgery. Neurosurgical Focus. 2012;**33**(5):E15. DOI: 10.3171/2012.7.FOCUS12181

[34] van Asch CJ, Luitse MJ, Rinkel GJ, van der Tweel I, Algra A, Klijn CJ. Incidence, case fatality, and functional outcome of intracerebral haemorrhage over time, according to age, sex, and ethnic origin: A systematic review and meta-analysis. Lancet Neurology. 2010;**9**(2):167-176. DOI: 10.1016/S1474-4422(09)70340-0

[35] Mendelow AD, Gregson BA, Fernandes HM, et al. Early surgery versus initial conservative treatment in patients with spontaneous supratentorial intracerebral haematomas in the International Surgical Trial in Intracerebral Haemorrhage (STICH): A randomised trial. Lancet. 2005;**365**(9457):387-397. DOI: 10.1016/S0140-6736(05)17826-X

Chapter 2

Perspective Chapter: Clinical Standard of a Geriatric Patient as a Virtual Target for Correction of Pharmacotherapy of Hypertension and Stroke in the Elderly

Aleksandr Urakov, Aleksandr Samorodov and Varvara Sokolova

Abstract

One of the unresolved geriatric problems in neuropharmacology remains the lack of specifically designed drugs and therapeutic and preventive measures for older adults with hypertension and/or stroke. In particular, there are no standards for virtual geriatric patients aged 65–70 years, 70–90 years, and over 90 years, as well as courses of pharmacotherapy for diseases in them. The fact is that modern drugs and standards of their use in the treatment of diseases are still traditionally focused on a virtual object, which represents a person of mature age weighing about 70 kg. Therefore, it is proposed to develop clinical standards appropriate for three groups of geriatric patients. The main characteristics of health status, hypertension and rehabilitation of elderly people after a stroke, as well as the peculiarities of pharmacodynamics and pharmacokinetics of drugs are given. It is hoped that the use of such virtual targets will optimize the adjustment of treatment of hypertension and stroke in elderly people and will reduce drug complications and polypragmasy.

Keywords: drug, course pharmacotherapy, polypragmasy, complications, elderly person, longevity, safety

1. Introduction

In recent decades, most countries of the world have experienced an "aging" of society, as, on the one hand, the number of elderly people has increased and, on the other hand, the number of children and youth has decreased. The reason for this phenomenon was the increase in the average life expectancy of people with a simultaneous decrease in their birth rate [1]. The significant increase in the number of elderly patients has led to an increase in the role of geriatric problems in health care and, in particular, in neurology, pharmacology, and pharmacy. The fact is that medicine, as an art of healing, was formed in a period when the bulk of patients consisted of people of young and mature age, because at that time, the average life expectancy of people did not exceed 30 years [2]. Moreover, patients over the age of 65 were a rarity for the bulk of physicians at the time the foundations of medicine were formed.

That is why the extant basics of therapeutic and surgical treatment of diseases mainly reflect the experience of successful medical treatment of people of young and mature age, but not of the elderly or long-lived. This is clearly demonstrated by the main mysteries of healing, which are reflected in the two most famous aphorisms of Hippocrates [3]:

1. Do no harm (*lat. Noli nocere*).

2. The doctor treats, nature heals (*Lat. Medicus curat, natura sanat*).

The essence of these aphorisms boils down to the following: despite the fact that the doctor prescribes treatment, it is still not the doctor who heals the patient, but nature that sustains his vitality. No one today is likely to argue that these aphorisms reflect the basic mysteries of healing, not of the elderly and the long-lived, but of the young and the mature. Today, they are guided equally by doctors who are adherents of traditional medicine and all sorts of "healers" and herbalists, relying on the methods of nontraditional and folk medicine [4]. Consequently, the extant medical standards of diagnosis and treatment of sick people reflect the state of health and readiness for self-recovery of people of young and mature age.

Analysis of the content of ancient medical treatises, including Hippocratic writings, convinces us that these standards reflect the experience of doctoring not all sick people, but only those of them who voluntarily sought medical care themselves, knowing that they would have to pay for it, and who were able to pay for the costs associated with diagnosis and treatment. In addition, it is important to emphasize that these medical diagnostic standards were developed without the use of most modern diagnostic technologies, and treatment standards did not include modern medications and technologies for their use [5]. In addition, the medical canons discussed were mostly relevant only to patients who believed in God, in the miraculous power of the healer they chose and the medicine they prescribed. At the same time, it is clear to us today that the healer himself successfully healed mostly people no older than 65 years of age, but people of young and mature age. Today, it is unlikely that anyone would argue with the fact that people of young and mature age fell ill, as a rule, by accident, and their illness was a short-term phenomenon. Obviously, the biblical truth that Christ healed many sick people, especially those who believed in him, applies to patients of young and mature age rather than to the elderly and long-lived [6, 7].

Therefore, diagnostic and therapeutic standards that have survived unchanged are suitable mainly for the treatment of people of young and mature age, and are of little use in the treatment of elderly patients. The fact is that aging leads to decrease of physical and mental activity of a human being, depletes reserves of all organs and systems of human body, and finally decreases disease resistance. Moreover, physical health, typical for a person of young and mature age, is not typical for patients older than 65. But as a person ages, it is natural that frailty and exhaustion progress, and diseases begin to take on a prolonged character. It is a bitter truth that man is mortal, and death is more likely in old age than in adulthood and youth.

A striking sign of old age in humans and animals is the wear of teeth, increased hardness of skeletal muscles, thickening of the walls of blood vessels, the appearance of cholesterol plaques in blood vessels, increased blood pressure, impaired blood supply to the brain and heart, as well as malignant neoplasms in various organs [8, 9]. Earlier the above mentioned manifestations of old age were rarely encountered in medical practice due to the fact that very few people lived to old age. Nowadays, due to the continuing "aging" of society, these manifestations of old age are more frequent and therefore require their resolution more often. It is becoming more and more evident that it is very important to be able to treat this or that disease not so much in people of young and mature age, but in the elderly and in long-lived people. At the same time, the progress of geriatric medicine is hindered by the absence of special "geriatric" drugs and medical standards for diagnosis and treatment of such "manifestations" of old age such as adentia, hypertension, stroke, ischemic heart disease, and myocardial infarction.

2. The modern virtual average patient as the medical standard mature patient without hypertension and stroke

Despite the fact that the modern practice of neurologists has replaced young and mature patients with elderly patients, "geriatric" standards of care have not yet been developed. Under these circumstances, when providing medical care to patients over the age of 65, physicians apply the same medical standard that they do when treating young and mature patients. It is true that doctors have remembered since college that the pharmacodynamics and pharmacokinetics of all medications depend on the health status, gender, and age of patients, so these factors must be taken into account. However, the existing medical standards inhibit the initiative of physicians because it does not contain specific recommendations for adjusting the diagnosis and treatment of elderly patients and long-livers with, in particular, hypertension and stroke [10, 11].

Nevertheless, when treating hypertension and stroke in the elderly, each neurologist compares the anatomical and functional features of each elderly patient with the features of a virtual average ("standard") patient of young and mature age. In doing so, the physician seeks to identify the difference between them independently in order to use it to "geriatricize" the treatment of the disease in the elderly patient. These skills are very important because currently they are the only ones that can help the physician find a successful solution to most of the geriatric problems that have accumulated in the medical-pharmaceutical field.

It is no secret that throughout the history of medicine and drug-making, the role of the average statistical patient has implied an average (virtual) person who was of average age (ranging from 18 to 65 years) [2, 12, 13]. In other words, it was not a person of advanced age by modern standards. Also implicit was the following: Although each patient represented either a man or a woman of childbearing age, the virtual standard person was assumed to represent something statistically average between a man and a woman (figuratively speaking, this patient represented the "middle" sex). Therefore, the role of this subject was not a girl and/or a woman during menstrual bleeding, fertilization, pregnancy, childbirth, and/or lactation.

To this we should add that in the opinion of pharmacists and healers, a standard virtual patient had an average statistical body structure, an average statistical state of health, and could unexpectedly "fall ill" and relatively quickly improve his health himself, more precisely—without doctors and without using traditional (or nontraditional) medicines. It was implied that the virtual standard patient had normal blood pressure, and also did not have a stroke, did not die either before or in the process of healing (i.e., conventionally speaking, lived "forever"). It was also assumed that the virtual standard patient had a body weight of about 70 kg, was not an alcoholic, drug addict, or substance abuser, had never previously taken any medications, had no drug addiction and led a daytime lifestyle, and ordinary diseases plagued him only during his waking period (namely, during the day) [7, 14].

On this basis, all generally accepted diagnostic and treatment standards (including pharmacological, pharmaceutical, and neurological technologies (diagnostic and treatment methods)), devices (medical instruments and devices), and means (drugs) are still not directly relevant to each specific person (patient) and not in each specific moment of his life. In particular, modern pharmacological, pharmaceutical, and neurological standards are relatively directly relevant only to those people of young and mature age (patients) who by the characteristics of their anatomo-functional state come close to the similar state of the virtual average patient currently accepted as a standard (conventional norm).

Thus, the main characteristics of the anatomical–functional state of the modern statistical average standard patient can be described by the following main indicators of his "nature": average age, average sex, average weight, and average state of health.

From this "rule," in particular, it follows that modern tablets of medicines are produced by pharmaceutical companies around the world with such mechanical, physical, chemical, and other properties, which are optimal for enteral administration in conditionally healthy people aged 18–65 years, who have intact chewing and speech apparatus and gastrointestinal tract. However, no one denies that modern drug tablets are prepared by pressing dry powders, so they are essentially quite strong artificial stones with varying hardness, which, by the way, is not controlled worldwide [15]. In this regard, it is no coincidence that pills, which are considered of high quality today, can cause local damage to the teeth, gums, and stomach walls not only in some patients, but also in healthy people. In this regard, there is reason to remind ourselves that man is not a bird. Humans are designed to swallow elastic, soft, and slippery chewing lumps, not hard stones [16].

Despite these paradoxes, tablets continue to be the top-selling drug among other dosage forms worldwide for the treatment of many diseases in people of all age groups, including the treatment of hypertension and stroke.

Under these conditions, in the complete absence of drugs produced in the form of special "geriatric" tablets, neurologists have no choice but to prescribe drugs to all elderly people in the form of the most common tablets, regardless of whether patients have teeth, dental prostheses, as well as the condition of the chewing and speech system and the gastrointestinal tract. At the same time, all physicians are informed that prescribing modern tablet medications strictly according to the accompanying "Instructions for Use" is correct only when treating people of young and mature age. Therefore, when prescribing medications in such "tablets" for the elderly and seniors, adjustments to the quality of the tablets, changes in the dose of the drugs they contain, and the technology of their enteral administration are required. However, pharmacological handbooks, instructions, and medication guidelines do not provide specific recommendations for turning "adult" pills into "geriatric" pills [17, 18]. The lack of precise instructions for neurologists on how to turn "adult" pills into "geriatric" pills does not optimize pharmacotherapy for diseases of the elderly, including the treatment of hypertension and stroke.

3. Basic geriatric syndromes and diseases—their importance in the treatment of hypertension and stroke in the elderly

The lack of "geriatric" drugs specifically designed to treat hypertension and stroke in elderly patients, as well as the progressive depletion of adaptation reserves to many diseases that occur with aging, predetermines the inevitable protracted nature of pathology and low efficiency of natural and/or medical rehabilitation of patients. Nevertheless, sometimes the patient's organism can retain some part of reserves and protective forces, which, for various reasons, are not involved in rehabilitation, but with the participation of a doctor can be used for this purpose. That is why in order to really improve the results of treatment of all patients, regardless of their age, all doctors must strive to unlock all available adaptation reserves of each patient to the fullest extent possible. That is why it is advisable to bring together as soon as possible all the accumulated positive experience in the treatment of hypertension and stroke in elderly and long-lived patients.

There is no doubt that elderly patients differ from young and mature patients in less reactivity of the body and a longer period of illness and rehabilitation after an illness. With increasing age, the reactivity of the body and the severity of its response not only to disease but also to drugs decreases. At the same time, aging leads to a decrease in the quality of life of people. Instead of the former curiosity, initiative desire to learn and succeed in learning observed in young years, in old age, people's craving for cognitive activity decreases. At the same time, such geriatric syndromes as senile asthenia, sarcopenia, depression, delirium, decreased skeletal-muscular mobility, and increased bone fragility, urinary incontinence, sensory deficits, oral disabilities (masticatory-speech apparatus dysfunction) develop [19–22].

It so happened that neurologists encountered difficulty in solving geriatric problems earlier than physicians in other specialties. This is explained by the fact that the increase in the average life expectancy of people first created the problem of high mortality and disability, which was caused by the increasing frequency of cardiovascular diseases. That is why neurology, cardiology, angiology, hematology, laboratory diagnostics, resuscitation, and anesthesiology and other allied medical specialties, including pharmacology and pharmacy, were developed at a rapid pace to address the above geriatric problems at that time. As a result, significant advances have been made in the prevention and medical treatment of hypertension, strokes, coronary heart disease, thrombosis, cardiopulmonary failure, and hypoxic cortical cell damage [23].

Only then, among other problems related to complications arising in the elderly from cardiovascular diseases, did the problems of rehabilitation of patients related to their musculoskeletal disorders begin to be developed. At the same time, the foundations for solving these geriatric problems were laid not in pharmacy and pharmacology, but in neurology. The fact is that initially, similar problems (paresis, paralysis, and even strokes) were often encountered in the practice of neurologists because they arose due to congenital, traumatic, ischemic, and/or hypoxic lesions of the brain cells in patients of young and mature age. In particular, thanks to neurologists, it has been conclusively proven that speech disorders are often a consequence not just of "old age," hypertension, and/or stroke, but rather of co-morbidities such as ischemic heart disease, diabetes, chronic lung, liver and kidney inflammation, and neurosurgical interventions. It has been shown that speech disorders can cause ischemic and/or hypoxic brain disorders, which, in turn, can manifest as aphasia and dysarthria, often combined with pathology of other higher mental functions (various types of agnosia and apraxia), impaired swallowing function, and motor and mental disorders (depression, severe neurotic states, and suicidal thoughts) [24–27]. Due to the efforts of neurologists and cardiologists, in recent years, some medications, in particular oral anticoagulants, have been additionally included in the list of causes of disability associated with provoking stroke, thrombosis, and bleeding [28].

Neurologists, through their established practice of collaborating with speech–language pathologists and physical therapists, have thoroughly investigated the effectiveness of various rehabilitation options for older patients with hypertension and stroke. The results they obtained allowed them to highlight the most effective methods and procedures. In particular, based on the experience of comprehensive rehabilitation of the masticatory-speech apparatus impaired in patients as a result of stroke and craniocerebral trauma, neurologists gave preference to the method of restorative training of patients [29–31].

It is noteworthy that aphasia, dysarthria, articulatory apraxia, speech, and swallowing disorders, encountered in the practice of neurologists when treating patients of young and mature age, were the consequence of local irreversible damage to the brain areas. And, as we know, dead brain cells do not regenerate. Today, however, it is becoming clear that rehabilitation based on teaching (training) of patients can accelerate the recovery of lost nervous system functions resulting from the death of some brain cells. The fact is that as a result of specially designed regular training, living neurons can take over the function of the damaged parts of the brain. Studies have shown that such training can often restore speech and swallowing function in patients of different ages. Therefore, the rehabilitation of the masticatory-speech apparatus of elderly patients can indeed be improved with restorative training, but not as quickly as one would like. Practice has shown that tangible rehabilitation success comes not earlier than after 3 to 6 weeks of regular training [32–36].

In parallel, neurologists have investigated the possibility of accelerating the process of rehabilitation of the masticatory-speech apparatus of elderly and senile patients with the help of medications. However, there was no convincing evidence of a significant increase in the effectiveness of the restorative teaching method. These results suggest that it is the method of restorative teaching that can be considered today as the basis of medical technology for the rehabilitation of the masticatory-speech apparatus in elderly patients who have suffered a stroke. Such "logopedic" rehabilitation can be based on regular (daily) theoretical and practical lessons with patients lasting 10–40 minutes each. Rehabilitation measures developed and tested in clinical practice include medication support, therapeutic gymnastics, speech therapy classes, massage, neuropsychological correction, and psychotherapeutic care. It is important to note that the success of these measures was achieved without the use of special "geriatric" medications.

In this case, it is implied that medical support for rehabilitation measures is reduced to the common course pharmacotherapy of the main and/or concomitant diseases, which may not refer only to neurological diseases. In turn, it is implied that pharmacotherapy of each disease should be carried out in accordance with the medical standard.

Stroke is one of the main diseases in elderly patients with rehabilitation measures aimed at restoring the function of the masticatory-speech apparatus. Since the cause of stroke may be craniocerebral trauma, hypertensive crisis, or cerebral vascular thrombosis, it is implied that medication support for speech rehabilitation of the masticatory-speech apparatus should be adjusted in full compliance with the available medication standards for craniocerebral trauma, hypertension, or hypercoagulation syndrome (or thromboembolic disease). In turn, comorbidities in patients of age and longevity can often be diabetes mellitus, chronic bronchitis, bronchial asthma, coronavirus infection, and some other diseases [37, 38]. Therefore, it is self-evident that in such cases, the medical support of the ongoing rehabilitation of the masticatory-speech apparatus should be adjusted (supplemented with drugs) in accordance with the standard of course pharmacotherapy of the relevant diseases and their complications (such as diabetic foot, airway obstruction, pulmonary emphysema, bilateral atypical pneumonia).

Consequently, the aging of the elderly person is most often manifested and/or accompanied by certain geriatric syndromes, which are mainly of a psychoneurological nature. Regardless of this, older people may often have concomitant diseases of various organs and systems of somatic nature. Therefore, medication support for stroke rehabilitation in the elderly cannot be standard and absolutely the same for all patients. In addition, it cannot be a monotherapy (therapy with a single drug). Proper medication support for stroke rehabilitation for each elderly patient must always be an original combination pharmacotherapy regimen in which the drugs must be carefully selected to take into account all the geriatric syndromes and illnesses of each individual patient.

4. Peculiarities of choice and prescription of drugs for the elderly in rehabilitation after stroke: Prevention of polypragmasy and its consequences

One of the unresolved geriatric problems in neurology remains the lack of "geriatric" medications and rehabilitation therapeutic and preventive measures designed exclusively for the elderly people and long-livers who have had a stroke. The lack of clinical standards for average patients of appropriate age groups (65–70, 70–90, and over 90 years old), geriatric medications, and geriatric regimens for course pharmacotherapy (drug support) of their rehabilitation after a stroke does not contribute to solving problems of geriatric neurology, especially in the treatment of hypertension and stroke.

Despite the unresolved geriatric problems, it is currently neurologists who are involved in the rehabilitation of elderly patients after stroke, as patients have traditionally sought medical care from neurologists for 160 years for this pathology. In this situation, doctors are forced to choose and prescribe medications for elderly and senile neurological patients on their own, doing so at their own risk. The fact is that neurologists have no right to refuse treatment to the elderly and long-term residents. Moreover, until today, all doctors are obliged to treat young, mature, and elderly patients equally, namely, in strict compliance with the medical standard, using traditional medications for this purpose.

However, when treating elderly people and long-livers (as opposed to young and mature patients), physicians need to combine medications more often, because elderly patients are more likely to have comorbidities. Because of this, physicians often have to use additional pharmacotherapy regimens. In particular, rehabilitation of elderly people after a stroke is often carried out against the background of geriatric syndromes of neuropsychiatric nature and diseases of various organs and systems of somatic nature. Moreover, aging of elderly patients reduces their reactivity, disease resistance, sensitivity to drugs, and the ability to inactivate the administered drugs [39, 40].

In these circumstances, to improve the effectiveness of pharmacotherapy and rehabilitation of geriatric patients, physicians are often forced to increase single, daily, and course doses of drugs, use new drugs and new drug combinations, expand the list of combined drugs and prescribe longer courses of pharmacotherapy. All this increases the risk of polypragmasy, side effects, drug complications, and poisoning; that is, it reduces the safety of drug therapy [39, 41, 42].

Many factors make this problem difficult to solve. First, an increase in the age of patients reduces their sensitivity to drugs (reduces the strength of the effect of drugs on the human body). This is caused, on the one hand, by a decrease in the reactivity of the organism as it ages, and on the other hand, by the development of addiction to drugs. At the same time, the decrease in the reactivity of the organism is universal and applies equally to many influences, including many drugs (also almost equally). Addiction to drugs is strictly individual in nature because it develops only in those patients who have previously used drugs for long courses. Moreover, in the case where drugs were used rarely, not regularly, and in short courses in adulthood, the use of drugs in old age may show no or very weak habituation to them, which may not be essential for the choice and prescription of drugs in the treatment of stroke in old age. In the other case, when drugs have been used frequently, regularly, and in long courses in adulthood, the use of drugs in old age may manifest itself by the presence of a strong habituation to them, which may deprive the action of these drugs or their analogues in the doses taken, but maintain their pharmacological activity when the single and/or daily doses are increased. It may be quite different when a person has been taking drugs at a young and/or mature age on a regular basis and for several months or years. The thing is that in this case, a person may develop drug addiction (drug disease) which is characterized by perversion of the effects of drug and development of withdrawal syndrome when the drug is withdrawn. The fact that the patient has drug dependence is confirmed by the development of withdrawal syndrome in the field of drug use cessation [28]. The presence of a patient's drug dependence requires a neurologist to consult a narcologist.

Second, as a rule, an increase in the age of patients is accompanied by a decrease in the intensity of their metabolism and inactivation of biologically active substances, including drugs. Therefore, with increasing age, the half-life of drugs (drug elimination half-life) usually increases in the elderly, the value of which is commonly indicated by the symbol $T_{1/2}$. By the way, in some elderly patients and in long-livers, the intensity of drug neutralization may be decreased not only because of the reduced intensity of general metabolism, but also because of the probable inhibition of the functional activity of the liver and kidneys. Therefore, to preserve the safety of course pharmacotherapy (to prevent chronic poisoning, i.e., to prevent overdose) in elderly patients, it is advisable to prescribe medications less frequently than indicated in the instructions for use of drugs, as these "instructions" currently apply only to patients of young and mature age. In addition, elderly patients are highly likely to have underlying or overt cardiovascular, liver, and kidney diseases. These diseases may be additional factors in slowing down the metabolism, inactivation, and/or excretion of drugs (and their metabolites) from the body [43, 44]. Therefore, the presence of hepatic, renal, and/or cardiovascular insufficiency in some patients contributes to an additional prolongation of the period of many drugs in the body, increasing the probability of their accumulation and overdose development during a long-course pharmacotherapy carried out with standard single doses and time intervals between their injections during drug rehabilitation of older patients who have had a stroke.

Third, the prescription of several drugs from different pharmacological groups to elderly patients simultaneously in the presence of geriatric syndromes of neuropsychiatric nature and diseases of various organs and systems of somatic nature predetermines the creation of an incredible multitude of combinations of different drugs with each other. The fact is that an average statistical patient today receives in different countries of the world during an average statistical course of pharmacotherapy 7–14 drugs. Moreover, more than half of them are prescribed simultaneously with each other [14]. At the same time, some of them are a ready combination of several drugs. At the same time, the characteristics of the pharmacodynamics and pharmacokinetics of the drugs in their combinations remain a mystery to most physicians in almost all specialties. Nevertheless, this unique information can be found by any physician if he opens the "white" book of pharmacology.

In this regard, a doctor who organizes medication support for rehabilitation of elderly stroke patients is likened to a kind of conductor of a drug orchestra, which under the doctor's control can play a certain "tune" in the patient's body. At the same time, the desired "sound" of the drug orchestra occurs only when each musician (in this case, when the effect of each drug is skillfully managed) plays skillfully. However, the mechanism of action of all possible combinations in the organism of an elderly patient is not described [7, 14, 18]. Therefore, a highly qualified physician and his ability to think philosophically are very important because only this can give the physician an understanding of the essence of combination pharmacotherapy. Only a philosopher doctor can manage the pharmacodynamics and pharmacokinetics of drugs when they are combined in the body of a particular elderly patient. The fact is that in a physician-uncontrolled drug combination, *no drugs, even the best ones, will ever 'play' a good tune together and produce nothing but "noise"* [14].

In daily therapeutic practice, most doctors who combine drugs fear side effects, complications, and overdose the most. The fact is that as a student, every doctor remembers Paracelsus' winged dictum "All things are poisons, for there is nothing without poisonous qualities. It is only the dose which makes a thing poisonous. This means that all things are poisons, for there is nothing without poisonous qualities. Only the dose makes a thing poisonous" [45]. A wise physician, therefore, when combining remedies, limits his choice to mildly and moderately active agents and their small doses, fearing as fire the remedies related to strongly active agents and poisons.

It has been reported that when it is necessary to use potent drugs for combination pharmacotherapy, in order to avoid complications and overdose, they should be used only in very low doses, namely in doses that are 1/10 to 1/20 of their usual therapeutic dose or even less [7, 14].

Nevertheless, the physician should always remember that the conditions of interaction of each drug with the body of each patient may change at any time of the pharmacotherapy. The most variable interaction factors are the patient's psychoemotional state, the value of temperature, humidity, ambient air, oxygen content in the breathing gas, total and local body temperature of the patient, the value of atmospheric pressure, the degree of illumination of the patient, his waking or sleeping state, and time of day. Moreover, the physician should assume that the conditions of interaction of drugs with the body of an elderly patient who has had a stroke will change the more likely and more significantly the longer the course of the ongoing pharmacotherapy will be.

5. Conclusion

In recent decades, in most countries of the world, the birth rate has decreased and life expectancy has increased significantly. Long-livers have appeared. In connection with this, the proportion of elderly people in society has increased, which has generally worsened the state of health in society, since the elderly fall ill more often than people of young and mature age. Hardly anyone would dispute the fact that aging leads to progressive "wear and tear" of the body, the fading of physical and mental activity, the depletion of the reserves of all organs and systems, and reduced resistance to disease. In this regard, older people are more often ill not only with diseases that occur at a young and mature age, but also with diseases caused by the aging (wear and tear) of the body. Therefore, elderly people and long-livers seek medical attention more often, and their diseases are prolonged and often combined with each other. Moreover, as the age of the elderly increases, their resistance to disease weakens. That is why the World Health Organization (WHO) recommends that physicians not only identify the elderly, but also divide them into three groups: patients aged 65–70 years, 70–90 years, and patients over 90 years (long-livers) [46].

These days, the health care system is not fully prepared to provide medical care to the elderly in all of these age groups. The fact is that the medical knowledge accumulated in the past and the established traditions of treating diseases (medical standards and medications) are oriented toward patients of young and mature age and are not oriented toward the elderly and long-term residents. Nevertheless, when treating the elderly, physicians are forced to use the same medical standards and medications as when treating the young and mature, because other medical standards and medications have not yet been developed.

Doctors know that diseases occur differently in older adults than in those who are young and mature, so doctors are prepared to make adjustments to their treatment, which should be the greater, the older the patient's age over 65. Physicians also know that traditional medical standards and medications are intended for use by patients of average age (18–65), average weight (weighing about 70 pounds), average gender, and average health (having sufficient reserves to recover independently from illnesses that occur by chance). This is the object recognized as the average patient today. Therefore, when treating an elderly patient, the doctor compares the anatomico-physiological features of his or her body condition with the corresponding parameters of the virtual (average) patient. If there is no significant difference, the doctor uses the medical standard without adjusting it, and if there is a significant difference, the doctor makes appropriate adjustments to the medical standard using special knowledge, the status of "treating physician," and the patient's legal right to informed consent.

However, not all physicians and not all cases manage to solve geriatric problems equally independently. The greatest difficulties in treating elderly patients arise for neurologists in the treatment of hypertension and stroke. It turns out that not only do neurologists lack appropriate geriatric medical standards and medications, but they also lack precise instructions on how to turn existing medical standards and medications into "geriatric" ones, especially when long-term rehabilitation of patients after a stroke is necessary.

Stroke is one of the most difficult diseases to treat in elderly patients. The fact is that in elderly patients, stroke and its consequences are often a consequence not only of hypertension, but also of such comorbidities as thromboembolic disease, coronary heart disease, diabetes mellitus, chronic pneumonia, liver, kidney, as well as neurosurgical intervention and course pharmacotherapy with oral anticoagulants. It has been shown that in stroke patients, the recovery of the lost functions of the nervous system can be accelerated by rehabilitation based on the training (coaching) of patients. For this purpose, special "speech therapy" rehabilitation measures were developed, including medication support, therapeutic gymnastics, massage, speech therapy classes, neuropsychological correction, and psychotherapeutic assistance. At the same time, medication support for the above rehabilitation measures in geriatric neurology was reduced to the common course pharmacotherapy not only for hypertension, but also for other comorbidities. As a result, the recommended drug support turned out to be essentially a combined pharmacotherapy of several diseases simultaneously. Moreover, today, this pharmacotherapy can be implemented in patients of all age groups only using the most common drugs, since there are no specially developed "geriatric" drugs.

It turned out that according to the established practice, neurologists are obliged to treat patients of young, mature, and elderly age according to a single medical standard, which relies exclusively on a diagnosis made without regard to the patient's age, and provides treatment of diseases through the use of traditional medications only. Because aging reduces the body's reactivity, resistance to disease, sensitivity to drugs, and ability to inactivate the drugs administered, when treating hypertension and/or stroke in the elderly, the physician in these circumstances is unwittingly in the role of an experimenter. The fact is that in these conditions, it is the neurologist who is forced to independently combine different medications and evaluate their effectiveness, because ready-made combined geriatric medications for the elderly and long-term patients have not yet been developed. The complexity of such a clinical trial is due to the fact that the combination of drugs may include 7–14 drugs from different pharmacological groups, and the combined pharmacotherapy lasts for many weeks and months in a row. In this case, the doctor is afraid not so much of the lack of therapeutic effect of the drugs prescribed by them, as of the damage caused by the drugs, since the combination of drugs is injected into a rather "worn out" organism.

So the lack of medical standards for averaged patients of appropriate age groups (65–70, 70–90, and over 90 years), special appropriate "geriatric" drugs and regimens for course pharmacotherapy of hypertension, stroke, and medical support for rehabilitation of elderly patients after a stroke hinders progress in geriatric neurology, pharmacology and pharmacy.

Can we today complement the only available virtual average patient's etalon reflecting the anatomical-functional state of a young and mature person with virtual patient's etalons reflecting the features of the anatomical-functional state of an average elderly person of the following age groups: 65–70, 70–90, and over 90 years old? Yes, of course, we can, because we have enough information about how the anatomico–functional state distinguishes the elderly from the young and the mature.

What would the development of such a clinical standard for the geriatric patient give us? Recognition of such a standard will ensure the development of a "geriatric" medical standard for diagnosis and treatment of diseases in older adults, "geriatric" medications, and "geriatric" regimens for combination pharmacotherapy of the most likely underlying and comorbidities (hypertension, stroke, diabetes mellitus, thromboembolic disease, coronary heart disease, atherosclerosis, chronic inflammation of the respiratory system, digestion, urinary tract, skin and external mucous membranes, arthrosis and arthritis, malignant neoplasms, etc.), which occur under conditions of reduced reactivity of the body, its resistance to disease, sensitivity to drugs, and the ability to inactivate the injected drugs. That is why the development of a clinical standard for the elderly patient aims at improving the diagnosis of diseases, increasing the efficiency and safety of treatment of the main group of modern patients, and reducing healthcare costs. In addition, it is hoped that the use of such virtual averaged elderly patients will optimize the adjustment of treatment of hypertension and stroke in the elderly, reducing drug complications and polypragmasy.

Conflict of interest

The author declares no conflict of interest.

Author details

Aleksandr Urakov[1*], Aleksandr Samorodov[2] and Varvara Sokolova[1]

1 Izhevsk State Medical University, Izhevsk, Russia

2 Bashkir State Medical University, Ufa, Russia

*Address all correspondence to: urakoval@live.ru

References

[1] National Research Council (US). Center for Economic, governance, and international studies. In: Grand Challenges of our Aging Society: Workshop Summary. Washington (DC): National Academies Press (US); 2010

[2] Donaldson L. Disease emergence and health transitions in the last millennium. Journal of the Royal College of Physicians of London. 2000;**34**(6):543-548

[3] Lloyd G, editor. Hippocratic Writings. 2nd ed. London: Penguin Books; 1983

[4] Amirdovlat A. Unnecessary for the Ignorant. Moscow: Science; 1990. (In Rus.)

[5] Nathanaël L, Guang-Biao Z, Bhavana P, Mitalic M, Zhue C, et al. Traditional knowledge-based medicine: A review of history, principles, and relevance in the present context of P4 systems medicine. Progress in Preventive Medicine. 2017;**2**(7):e0011. DOI: 10.1097/pp9.0000000000000011

[6] Святое Евангелие с толкованием святых отцов. The Holy Gospel as Interpreted by the Holy Fathers. Moscow: Syntagma; 2010. (In Rus.)

[7] Urakov AL. How drugs work inside us. Izhevsk: Udmurtia; 1993 (In Rus.)

[8] Khan SS, Singer BD, Vaughan DE. Molecular and physiological manifestations and measurement of aging in humans. Aging Cell. 2017;**16**(4):624-633. DOI: 10.1111/acel.12601

[9] Krut'ko VN, Dontsov VI, Khalyavkin AV, Markova AM. Natural aging as a sequential poly-systemic syndrome. Frontiers in Biosciences (Landmark Ed). 2018;**23**(5):909-920. DOI: 10.2741/4624

[10] Powers WJ, Rabinstein AA, Ackerson T, et al. Guidelines for the early Management of Patients with Acute Ischemic Stroke: A guideline for healthcare professionals from the American Heart Association/American Stroke Association [published correction appears in stroke]. Stroke. 2018;**49**(3):e46-e110. DOI: 10.1161/STR.0000000000000158

[11] Winstein CJ, Stein J, Arena R, et al. Guidelines for adult stroke rehabilitation and recovery: A guideline for healthcare professionals from the American Heart Association/American Stroke Association. Stroke. 2016;**47**(6):e98-e169. DOI: 10.1161/STR.0000000000000098

[12] Federspiel C, Keipes M. La Gériatrie du 19ième au 21ième siècle [geriatrics from the 19th to the 21st century. 150 years of geriatric medicine: From increasing life expectancy to improving quality of life for the very old]. Bull Soc Sci Med Grand Duche Luxemb. 2014:69-78

[13] Arai H, Ouchi Y, Toba K, et al. Japan as the front-runner of super-aged societies: Perspectives from medicine and medical care in Japan. Geriatrics & Gerontology International. 2015;**15**(6):673-687. DOI: 10.1111/ggi.12450

[14] Urakov AL. Basics of Clinical Pharmacology. Izhevsk Printing Works: Izhevsk; 1997

[15] Urakov A, Urakova N, Reshetnikov A, Kasatkin A, Kopylov M, Baimurzin D. About what is happening in the stomach after swallowing human river pebbles,

gravel, chalk, clay and tablets drugs. Epitőanyag–Journal of Silicate Based and Composite Materials. 2016;**68**(4):110-113. DOI: 10.14382/epitoanyag-jsbcm.2016.19

[16] Urakov AL. Tablet as a pharmaceutical form of medicinal products intended for administration inside: Advantages and disadvantages. Reviews on Clinical Pharmacology and Drug Therapy. 2018;**16**(3):13-18. DOI: 10.17816/RCF16313-18

[17] Ritter RJ, Flower RJ, Henderson G, Flower RJ. Rang & Dale's Pharmacology. Eighth ed. Churchill Livingstone; 2016

[18] Katzung BG, Vanderah TW, editors. Basic & Clinical Pharmacology. Fourteenth ed. San Francisco: McGraw Hill; 2021

[19] Inouye SK, Studenski S, Tinetti ME, Kuchel GA. Geriatric syndromes: Clinical, research, and policy implications of a core geriatric concept. Journal of the American Geriatrics Society. 2007;**55**(5):780-791. DOI: 10.1111/j.1532-5415.2007.01156.x

[20] Arai H, Ouchi Y, Yokode M, et al. Toward the realization of a better aged society: Messages from gerontology and geriatrics. Geriatrics & Gerontology International. 2012;**12**(1):16-22. DOI: 10.1111/j.1447-0594.2011.00776.x

[21] Schwab WS. Geriatric syndromes. Journal of the American Geriatrics Society. 2008;**56**(2):363-364. DOI: 10.1111/j.1532-5415.2007.01488.x

[22] Janac S, Clarke B, Gems D. Aging: Natural or disease? A view from medical textbooks. In: Vaiserman AM, editor. Anti-Aging Drugs: From Basic Research to Clinical Practice. Cambridge (UK): Royal Society of Chemistry; 2017

[23] Karenberg A. Historic review: Select chapters of a history of stroke. Neurological Research and Practice. 2020;**2**:34. DOI: 10.1186/s42466-020-00082-0

[24] Chen X, Mao G, Leng SX. Frailty syndrome: An overview. Clinical Interventions in Aging. 2014;**9**:433-441. DOI: 10.2147/CIA.S45300

[25] Rofes L, Arreola V, López I, Martin A, Sebastián M, Ciurana A, et al. Effect of surface sensory and motor electrical stimulation on chronic poststroke oropharyngeal dysfunction. Neurogastroenterology and Motility: the Official Journal of the European Gastrointestinal Motility Society. 2013;**25**(11):888-e701. DOI: 10.1111/nmo.12211

[26] de Sire A, Giachero A, de Santi S, Inglese K, Solaro C. Screening dysphagia risk in 534 older patients undergoing rehabilitation after total joint replacement: A cross-sectional study. European Journal of Physical and Rehabilitation Medicine. 2021;**57**(1):131-136. DOI: 10.23736/S1973-9087.20.06321-2

[27] Öner A, Abdullah S, Yenal K, Ömer D, Mahmut T. Intoxications: Why suicide ?, why women ? The Journal of Neurobehavioral Sciences. 2019;**6**(2):83-86. DOI: 10.5455/JNBS.1545649959

[28] Urakov A, Stolyarenko A, Yagudin I, Muhutdinov N, Bashirov I. Stroke, thrombosis, bleeding and addiction to anticoagulants in the context of course therapy: A pharmacologic perspective. Reviews in Cardiovascular Medicine. 2022;**23**(7):236. DOI: 10.31083/j.rcm2307236

[29] Almhdawi KA, Mathiowetz VG, White M, delMas RC. Efficacy of occupational therapy task-oriented

approach in upper extremity post-stroke rehabilitation. Occupational Therapy International. 2016;**23**(4):444-456. DOI: 10.1002/oti.1447

[30] Murrell JE, Pisegna JL, Juckett LA. Implementation strategies and outcomes for occupational therapy in adult stroke rehabilitation: A scoping review. Implementation Science. 2021;**16**(1):105. DOI: 10.1186/s13012-021-01178-0

[31] Zhang J, Yu J, Bao Y, et al. Constraint-induced aphasia therapy in post-stroke aphasia rehabilitation: A systematic review and meta-analysis of randomized controlled trials. PLoS One. 2017;**12**(8):e0183349. DOI: 10.1371/journal.pone.0183349

[32] Liu K, Zhang W, Yang Y, Zhang J, Li Y, Chen Y. Respiratory rehabilitation in elderly patients with COVID-19: A randomized controlled study. Complementary Therapies in Clinical Practice. 2020;**39**:101166. DOI: 10.1016/j.ctcp.2020.101166

[33] Di Marco R, Rubega M, Lennon O, et al. Experimental protocol to assess neuromuscular plasticity induced by an exoskeleton training session. Methods and Protocols. 2021;**4**(3):48. DOI: 10.3390/mps4030048

[34] Swank C, Trammell M, Bennett M, et al. The utilization of an overground robotic exoskeleton for gait training during inpatient rehabilitation-single-center retrospective findings. International Journal of Rehabilitation Research. 2020;**43**(3):206-213. DOI: 10.1097/MRR.0000000000000409

[35] McGlinchey MP, James J, McKevitt C, Douiri A, McLachlan S, Sackley CM. The effect of rehabilitation interventions on physical function and immobility-related complications in severe stroke-protocol for a systematic review. Systematic Reviews. 2018;**7**(1):197. DOI: 10.1186/s13643-018-0870-y

[36] Chen J, Or CK, Chen T. Effectiveness of using virtual reality-supported exercise therapy for upper extremity motor rehabilitation in patients with stroke: Systematic review and meta-analysis of randomized controlled trials. Journal of Medical Internet Research. 2022;**24**(6):e24111. DOI: 10.2196/24111

[37] Corlateanu A, Stratan I, Covantev S, et al. Asthma and stroke: A narrative review. Asthma Research and Practice. 2021;7:3. DOI: 10.1186/s40733-021-00069-x

[38] GBD 2019 Stroke Collaborators. Global, regional, and national burden of stroke and its risk factors, 1990-2019: A systematic analysis for the global burden of disease study 2019. Lancet Neurology. 2021;**20**(10):795-820. DOI: 10.1016/S1474-4422(21)00252-0

[39] Oganov R, Drapkina O. Polymorbidity: Specifics of co-development and concomitance of several diseases in one patient. Cardiovascular Therapy and Prevention. 2016;**15**:4-9. DOI: 10.15829/1728-8800-2016-4-4-9

[40] Mosconi MG, Paciaroni M. Treatments in ischemic stroke: Current and future. European Neurology. 2022;**85**(5):349-366. DOI: 10.1159/000525822

[41] Pazan F, Wehling M. Polypharmacy in older adults: A narrative review of definitions, epidemiology and consequences. European Geriatric Medicine. 2021;**12**(3):443-452. DOI: 10.1007/s41999-021-00479-3

[42] Novak J, Goldberg A, Dharmarajan K, et al. Polypharmacy in older adults with cancer undergoing

radiotherapy: A review. Journal of Geriatric Oncology. 2022;**13**(6):778-783. DOI: 10.1016/j.jgo.2022.02.007

[43] Schlender JF, Meyer M, Thelen K, et al. Development of a whole-body physiologically based pharmacokinetic approach to assess the pharmacokinetics of drugs in elderly individuals. Clinical Pharmacokinetics. 2016;**55**(12):1573-1589. DOI: 10.1007/s40262-016-0422-3

[44] Cui C, Valerie Sia JE, Tu S, et al. Development of a physiologically based pharmacokinetic (PBPK) population model for Chinese elderly subjects. British Journal of Clinical Pharmacology. 2021;**87**(7):2711-2722. DOI: 10.1111/bcp.14609

[45] Grandjean P. Paracelsus revisited: The dose concept in a complex world. Basic & Clinical Pharmacology & Toxicology. 2016;**119**(2):126-132. DOI: 10.1111/bcpt.12622

[46] Lee SB, Oh JH, Park JH, Choi SP, Wee JH. Differences in youngest-old, middle-old, and oldest-old patients who visit the emergency department. Clinical and Experimental Emergency Medicine. 2018;**5**(4):249-255. DOI: 10.15441/ceem.17.261

Chapter 3

Clinical Usefulness of Real-time Sensory Compensation Feedback Training on Sensorimotor Dysfunction after Stroke

Takayuki Kodama and Ken Kitai

Abstract

The sensory dysfunction after the stroke also greatly affects motor function. In particular, it is known that the presence of sensory dysfunction in the fingers causes loss of somatosensory muscle reflex control and excessive muscle output when grasping objects. These are called sensorimotor dysfunction and have been shown to have a significant impact on prognosis. One element to improve this dysfunction is to reconstruct the "Sense of Agency (SOA) subject feeling" and it has become clear that SOA is enhanced by matching the collation information related to motor intention and sensory feedback in time. In order to reconstruct the SOA associated with the movement of the fingers of patients with sensorimotor dysfunction, it is important to match motor intentions while using visual information as compensation for tactile sensory information. Furthermore, considering the functional characteristics of the fingers, it is also important to adjust the fine muscle output from feedback information synchronously discriminating and recognizing somatosensory information generated by resistance, friction, etc., when an object is actively touched. This chapter outlines the importance of rehabilitation of sensory feedback for poststroke sensorimotor dysfunction and investigates the usefulness of intervention with a real-time sensory compensation feedback system that can input tactile sensory information via vibratory stimulation (deep sensation) to other body parts where sensory function is preserved.

Keywords: stroke, rehabilitation, sensorimotor dysfunction, neurofeedback, sensory feedback, sense of agency, EEG

1. Introduction

Stroke is one of the main diseases that cause sequelae disorders [1], typically including chronic sensory and motor dysfunction in the body [2]. These disorders are often not isolated but occur in combination with poststroke sensorimotor impairment (PSI). PSI in the hand, in particular, has a significant impact on functional disability, behavior, lifestyle [3], and quality of life (QOL) [4]. PSI limits the scope of the exercises and activities an individual can perform and is a factor in the degree of reliance on caregivers. One approach to this is neurorehabilitation. Neurorehabilitation is a concept or intervention approach that seeks to improve disability through interdisciplinary interventions that include physiotherapy. For successful rehabilitation of patients with different symptoms, it is important to identify the causative mechanisms of the disability and implement an individually optimized approach [5]. For this reason, it is important to input sensory feedback information properly in relation to motor images and intentions, without any time lag [6]. As a result, the sense of agency (SOA), which is one of the elements of body awareness, —'it is you yourself who moves your hand,'—increases and motor learning advances [7]. Since the primary motor cortex (M1) and coordinated activities in the parietal cortex area are involved in the SOA [8], enhancing the SOA may improve hand function by activating the nervous system for motor control centered in the corticospinal tract. However, there are no established treatments for PSI of the hand based on these perspectives, and improving hand dexterity remains a difficult task. This paper summarizes the impact of hand PSI on the body and mind and the approaches taken to date; further, the effectiveness of an intervention using a real-time feedback system for tactile perception discrimination as a new approach is discussed.

2. Concept of sensory disturbance as a sequela of stroke

Stroke is a general term for a disease in which the function of the brain is impaired due to abnormalities in the blood vessels in the brain. Blood clots form in the brain, blocking blood flow, clogging arteries, breaking blood vessels, and causing bleeding. If the myriad arteries in the brain rupture, the lack of oxygen leads to the sudden death of brain cells. Most strokes (87%) are ischemic infarctions [9]. Stroke is the second leading cause of death worldwide and the third leading cause of residual disability due to its severe impact on the brain and a large number of cases. The incidence of stroke increases with age, doubling after 55 years of age. However, in an alarming trend, between 1990 and 2016, strokes among people aged 20–54 years increased from 12.9% to 18.6% of all cases worldwide. Nevertheless, age-standardized cause mortality decreased by 36.2% in the same period [10]. All this means that while the rates of lives saved are increasing due to developments in medical care, the number of people with poststroke sequelae are also increasing. Additionally, it means that the socioeconomic burden of stroke patients with sequelae is increasing over time [11]. Therefore, despite advances in stroke management, poststroke care has a significant impact on families, the health system, and the economy. Thus, improvements in preclinical and clinical care may support not only the primary treatment of stroke but also successful recovery, rehabilitation, and prevention of sequelae. Therefore, stroke management systems need to include physiotherapy approaches in addition to existing primary care, as well as postdischarge occupational therapy and follow-up at poststroke care facilities.

One of the most serious sequelae after a stroke is hemiplegia, which consists of motor and sensory paralysis. Hemiplegia is a typical neurologically altered condition that can lead to physical and mental disability and affect daily living and quality of life. Therefore, 25–50% of stroke survivors require some form of assistance after discharge from the hospital. It is estimated that only 14% can recover sufficiently to perform activities of daily living [12]. While it is well known that motor paralysis affects motor function, sensory dysfunction of the upper extremities is also impaired in approximately 50–80% of adults after stroke, significantly limiting their ability to use the upper extremities [13–15]. This is poststroke sensorimotor impairment (PSI). Since these impairments not only interfere with sensory input but also diminish the use of the paralyzed upper extremity, PSI patients receive less sensorimotor information in daily life and are also more susceptible to factors such as vision, attention, and active awareness of working with objects [16]. Since they are constantly in this state, their attribution strategy can change, possibly resulting in misattribution even in the performance of the unparalyzed upper limb [17]. These factors make an approach to PSI, especially of the upper extremities, an important factor in constructing rehabilitation programs that improve the physical function and living ability of stroke patients.

3. Post-stroke sensorimotor impairment (PSI)

To date, most studies on upper limb motor function and recovery after stroke have been discussed in terms of brain plasticity. With normal brain function, upper limb movements the brain functional areas that govern them have a contralateral relationship, but after stroke this contralateral dominance pattern changes within a few weeks and the left-right difference decreases [18]. The poststroke period is characterized by activity in both hemispheres, and increased neural activity in the entire motor-related area has been reported [19]. In patients with right hemiplegia, brain activity associated with movement of the right upper extremity showed increased mobilization of the left dorsal premotor cortex (PM) and bilateral supplementary motor areas (SMA), in addition to shifting to the right hemisphere motor-related region (**Figure 1**). Moreover, the probability of mobilization of bilateral neural activity in many motor-related areas increases with the severity of paralysis [20], and the grip strength of the paralyzed hand is associated with the size of the motor-related cortical map being mobilized.

Accurate movement execution requires preparation, execution, and monitoring mechanisms based on network neural activity centered in the frontal lobe, parietal lobe, basal ganglia, and cerebellum, as well as motor-related areas [21]. Preparation and execution are performed by activation of the motor-related area systems, such as SMA and PM, to generate the preparatory potentials and preactivation of peripheral muscles necessary for purposeful exercise. The monitoring mechanism is the detection of sensory errors by the cerebellum and basal ganglia from the actual sensory input (feedback model) and the sensory information (forward model) predicted in advance. That error information is transmitted to the primary sensory cortex (S1), SMA, and PM. M1 receives the motor plans from the SMA and PM and generates the efference copy information, which is the basis of the forward model, and it constantly transmits to the parietal association area for comparison with the sensory feedback information. The sensorimotor integrative loop for enaction is the series of steps that must work properly to enable synaptic movement (**Figure 2**) [21]. This enables purposeful movements. The breakdown of these loops provokes unintentional involuntary movements. Therefore, while motor-related areas are strongly involved in muscle exertion in gross motor activities, such as grip strength, somatosensory areas are more active in the performance of skillful fine motor movements with the hands. In fact, by inputting the somatosensory information of the hand, the somatosensory area accurately represents the shape of the hand in the brain, integrates the necessary motor commands, and performs the selective activation of the muscles necessary for activities such as manipulating objects [22].

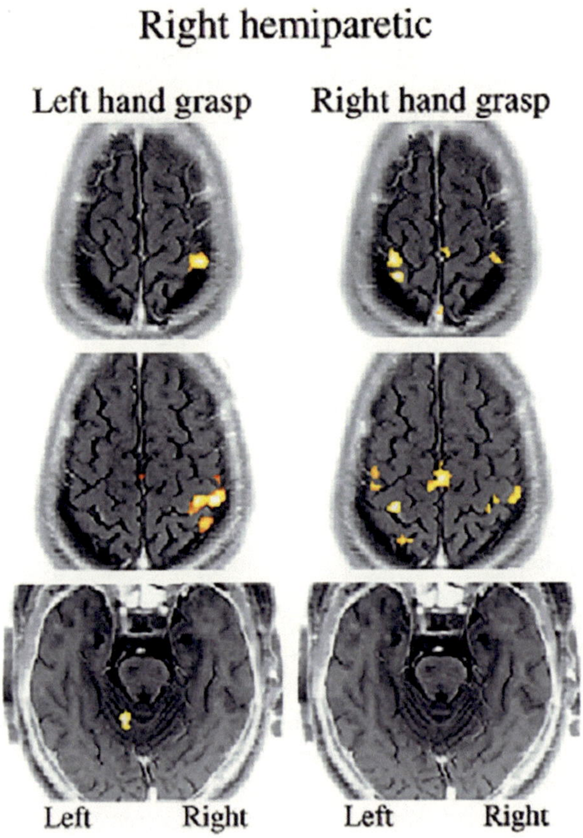

Figure 1.
In patients with post-stroke right hemiparesis, grasping movements of the paralyzed hand (right hand) showed a lateral shift of the motor cortex to the right hemisphere and increased neuromobilization of the left dorsal premotor cortex and bilateral supplementary motor cortex [19].

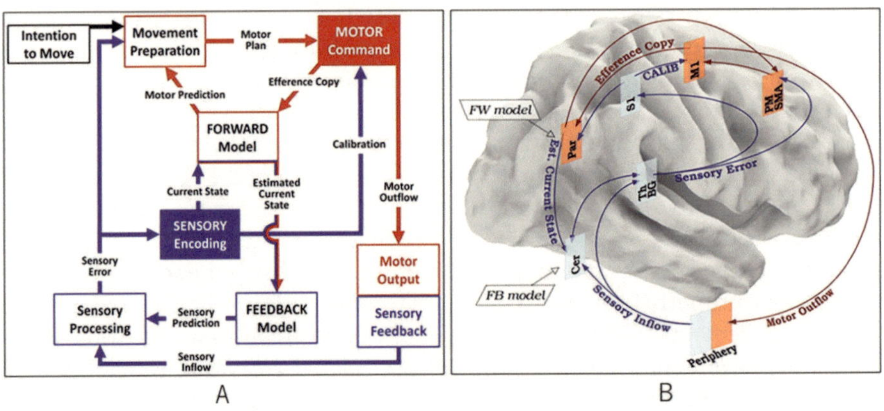

Figure 2.
Schematic diagram of the sensorimotor integrative loop for enacting (A) and the biological brain basis (B) [21]. The blue arrows indicate the flow of sensory feedback information, and the red arrows indicate the flow of forward information such as motor command, motor plan, and efference copy. In particular, the efference copy is an important element for comparing and predicting the kinaesthetic (forward model) and somatosensory (feedback model) consequences.

This suggests that if sensory information from the hands is not inputted into the brain, the selective activation of muscles needed for skillful movements may not occur, thereby causing problems in using the hands for movements such as using tools or buttoning a shirt. PSI of the hand caused by this sensory dysfunction has been reported to result from damage to the central nervous system's afferent pathways, such as the somatosensory area [23]. When these symptoms appear, the ability to perform the activities of daily living is greatly reduced and daily life becomes difficult [24]. Doyle et al. [13] reviewed 13 reports of various treatment interventions for upper extremity sensory impairment in 467 participants. They found that only two studies examined each specific intervention. and in many cases, there was insufficient evidence to support or refute their effectiveness in improving participants' functional status and participation. Therefore, they indicated the need for more appropriately designed and better-reported sensory rehabilitation studies. To solve these problems, it is necessary to grasp the sequence of the information processing mechanisms between the hand and the brain for somatosensory information to be connected to movement, from a neurological perspective, and put the elements required for that into the conditions of the intervention technique.

4. Effects of sensorimotor disorders on the hand

4.1 Neurological functioning of the hand

When manipulating an object, humans have a variety of inputs from tactile afferents in the hand to the brain, including the time course, magnitude, direction, and spatial distribution of contact forces, the shape of the contact surface (texture, roughness, softness, etc.), and friction between the contact surface and the fingers [25, 26]. To skillfully capture such tactile information, Meissner bodies, Merkel cells, Ruffini endings, and Pacinian corpuscles are located in the finger pads. These tactile afferents classify mechanical stimuli from the viewpoints of adaptation and receptive fields (**Figure 3A**); however, FA-II (40–400 Hz), which is predominantly Pacinian corpuscles, is sensitive to dynamic skin deformations at relatively high frequencies, and SA-II, which is mainly Ruffini corpuscles, is most readily excited by low-frequency skin deformation and can respond to sustained deformations [27]. FA-II and SA-II afferent nerves innervate the hand with a low and almost uniform density, ending deeper in the dermis and subcutaneous fibrous tissue. Hundreds of FA-II afferent nerves, distributed throughout the hand, increase neural excitation when the hand contacts or breaks contact with an object. SA-II afferent nerves, in contrast, respond to remotely applied lateral stretching of the skin and are sensitive to tangential shear strain to the skin that occurs during object manipulation [28, 29]. These sensory receptors are capable of discriminating differences in roughness and friction in detail (**Figure 3B**).

Therefore, it is possible to input information in response to various friction coefficients generated between the hand and the object due to the difference in spatial frequency characteristic information that can be captured. When humans manipulate an object, they need to hold the object statically and react and control the sharp friction generated in the finger pad. In particular, the function of the Pacinian corpuscle, which corresponds to the spatial frequency range from the micro to macro levels, plays an important role in hand control. It is a vibration that creates these spatial frequencies. Vibrations caused by friction are transmitted to

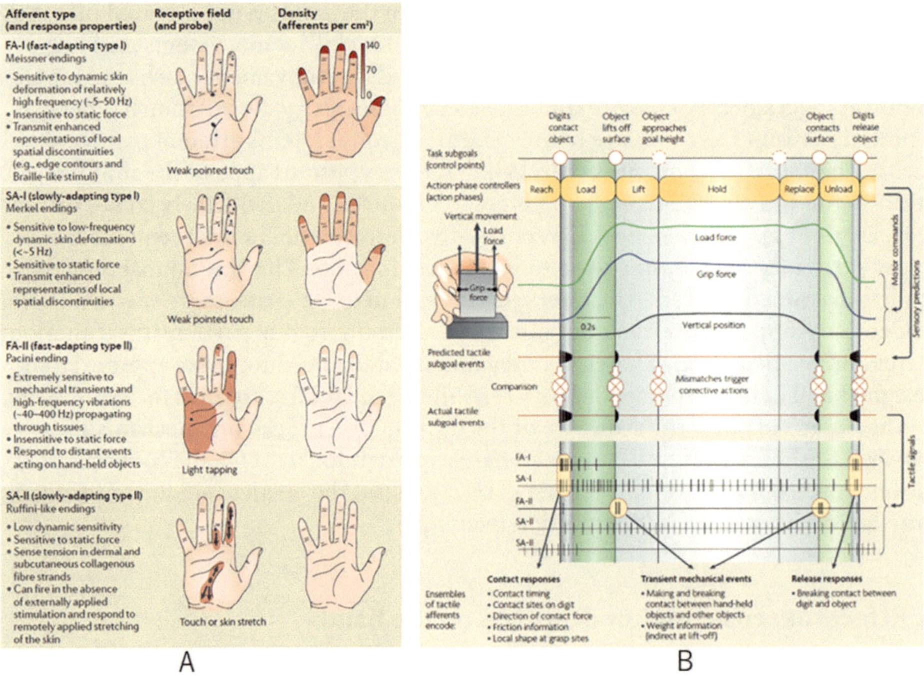

Figure 3.
Tactile innervation of the fingers (A) and sensorimotor control points in an object manipulation task (B) [26]. A: The inside of the human hand is equipped with four functionally district types of tactile afferents. B: Finger-object contact corresponds to a discrete sensory event characterized by the involvement of specific afferent nerves.

tactile receptors in the finger pad, and signals from the tactile receptors i.e., feedback information corresponding to hand movements, are inputs to the brain [30]. By detecting friction information generated when the hand touches the object through this process, the brain controls the force of the fingertip to avoid slipping, and this brain control system makes it possible to manipulate the object without dropping it [31]. Therefore, when considering rehabilitation for PSI after a stroke, it is necessary to compensate for the inputting of the frictional information sensed by the hand as somatosensory information, which is controlled in the brain and converted into execution of movement. This is thought to be important for the reorganization of sensorimotor functioning.

4.2 Problems caused by PSI in the hand

It is known that a decreased sense of belonging for one's own hand due to PSI induces a symptom called learned nonuse, in which the affected hand does not participate in the activities of daily living, independent of the degree of motor dysfunction [32]. This greatly reduces the abilities involved in the activities of daily living [33]. Despite good movement ability, survivors of sensory loss learn not to use their hands to perform tasks [34]. Thus, Carey et al. [35] reported that the somatosensory impairment status poststroke while hospitalized was associated with more loss of participation in activities in the absence of concomitant paralysis, compared with survivors without somatosensory loss. This predictive association was confirmed in a longitudinal cohort (N = 268) study of stroke survivors with mild disabilities. Additionally,

PSI has a significant impact on quality of life [36]. All of this suggests that in patients with neurological disease who lose one or more senses the impact on their motor function may be serious, even if their muscle strength is not affected. After a stroke recovery of movement depends on the degree of sensory impairment [37]. Against this background, rehabilitation aimed at restructuring motor function may decrease the outcome of functional recovery in stroke patients unless it encompasses intervention for sensory impairment. Historically, however, clinicians and researchers have prioritized the motor sequelae of stroke and ignored somatosensory impairment [38]. This may be because symptoms arising from sensory disorders are more varied and often rely on the patient's subjective information, in contrast to motor dysfunctions, which can be objectively measured.

If sensory feedback information continues to be properly inputted through the body, top-down control that allows for quick and continuous movement can be achieved. When humans perform exercises and movements, the brain extracts and integrates sensory information on the body position that accompanies them. Concurrently, the body's future sensory state is estimated from motor commands based on higher-order top-down forward information such as memories, intentions, and intentions regarding previous experience and skills. These brain processing systems enable the activation of a predictive mechanism, called the internal forward model, that suppresses predicted sensory feedback [37, 39]. This top-down control, based on motor imagery and SOA, is largely the function of M1, an output mechanism to the corticospinal tract [40]. By utilizing this top-down control, humans can continually minimize the displacement of slip, when the hand contacts an object, without relying on sensory feedback information. Additionally, top-down control is constructed by continuous synchronous and sensitive feedback of friction information, e.g., vibration stimulus information inputs from the sensory receptors of the fingers to the brain, which is generated when the hand touches an object. Therefore, in rehabilitation, it is important to have an approach that enables continuous feedback of hand-touch friction information in a synchronous and precise manner. However, since it is difficult for PSI patients to precisely grasp sensory information from their hands, it is crucial to construct an approach theory that provides them with compensatory input stimuli and enhances their learning efficiency.

4.3 PSI of the hand and transformation of body awareness

Body awareness is self-body recognition and is the brain's systemic basis for motor development. This ability enables humans to recognize differences between themselves and others, as well as between themselves and the outside world, and to adapt their bodies to their environment. It has been reported that body awareness causes schizophrenic-like symptoms, such as hands that feel alien, like someone else's hands, or that someone is inserting such thoughts [41]. Gallagher et al. [41] have shown that it is important to have a "minimal self" to activate body awareness. The minimal self is the "immediate awareness of oneself as a body" through daily exercise and life experience. There is no need for oneself to be aware of that here. This allows for the identification of two separate modalities: the sense of ownership (SOO), which states that one's body is oneself, and the SOA, which states that one is the one running one's body.

SOO is explained by a phenomenon called the rubber hand illusion [42]. This phenomenon is an illusion in which an inanimate rubber hand feels like one's own hand. The illusion is induced by blocking the visual information of the rubber hand and the patient's actual hand and stimulating tactile information to the skin synchronously (misalignment is within a few hundred milliseconds). This suggests that human body recognition can be altered by a specific stimulus presentation, which is a vital discovery for the study of human body awareness. The sensation of possessing a rubber hand is accompanied by a change in hand position sense (proprioception), therefore, when patients are asked to indicate the location of their (invisible) hand, they indicate that it is near the rubber hand. This is known as intrinsic receptive drift and is the most widely used objective measure of the rubber hand illusion, suggesting a close relationship between intrinsic receptivity and a sense of body ownership [43]. This sense of physical ownership is generated by the integrated processing of somatosensory and visual information within the parietal lobe [44], and it has been reported that alterations in the sense of body ownership, for example, tend to produce illusions and phantom limb pain in limb amputees [45].

In contrast, an SOA is a basis for the creation of cooperative neural network activity in the prefrontal cortex [46] and, in addition to M1 [8], the insular cortex (especially the anterior regions), lower parietal lobe regions (supramarginal and angular gyri), anterior cingulate gyrus of the cortical midline structure, supplementary motor cortex, posterior cingulate gyrus, and precuneus of the cortical midline structure are involved in the formation and the establishment [47]. The comparative matching of motor intention and sensory feedback information is generated by synchronous processing in the brain [7], and the sense of subjectivity diminishes with a temporal lag (**Figure 4**) [48]. Previous studies have also shown that an SOA is created if the misalignment is within 500 ms [49].

The following four explanatory models and concepts can be used to explain the SOA:

1. Time axis of the predictive and postdictive processes.

2. Axis of awareness of the explicit and implicit levels.

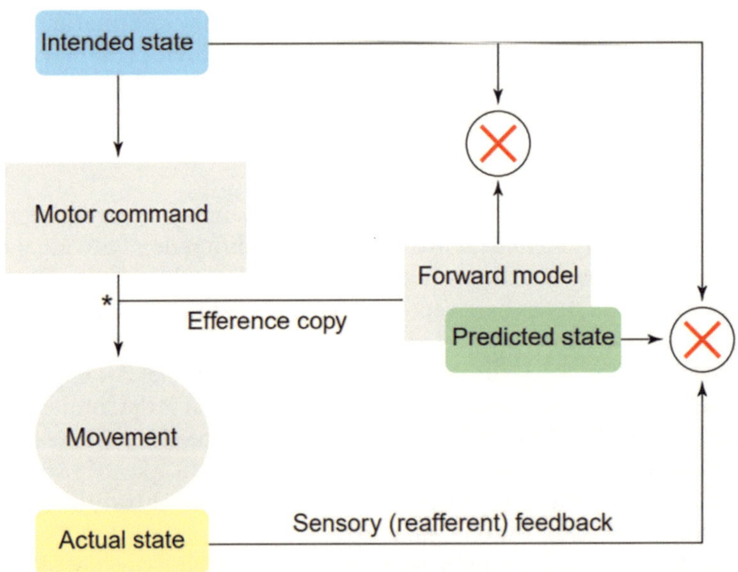

Figure 4.
The forward and feedback comparators [43]. Agreement in the forward comparator provides motor subjectivity to the movement.

3. Directed axes called internal cue and external cue.

4. A learning perspective that the sense of subjectivity is continually being renewed.

Point (1) is a perspective that includes a forecasting model. In general, an SOA is only a part of the self-consciousness associated with the act and is a feeling that can only be experienced after the act, but it can be modified by the postprocess, such as rewards obtained as a result of the act. Point (2) is a view of the hierarchy of conscious (conscious) and subconscious (unconscious) processes. Point (3) is that the SOA is supposed to be established based on various internal and external cues. Internal cues include intentions, objectives, plans, goals, predictive signals, priming, beliefs, knowledge, effort, and expectations of reward, while external cues include the effects of the action, contextual information, and rewards. The optimal SOA is based on the availability and reliability of each. The last point (4) is taken in terms of larger dynamics but is meant to be taken from the perspective of learning, where mechanisms such as these are not innate and fixed, but constantly updating as humans survive and adapt to their environment.

Furthermore, Synofzik et al. [50] state that an SOA exists hierarchically, with sensory and cognitive levels. An SOA generated by the temporal matching of information on movement intention and sensory feedback, as described above, is the feeling of agency (FOA) at the sensory level. Meanwhile, judgment of agency (JOA) is generated at the cognitive level when conceptual reasoning about discrimination of action types is processed and the status of SOA is made conscious in a form that can be verbalized. Therefore, it has been reported that even if the one executing a movement is the person himself or herself and if the actual sensory outcome deviates from the prediction, it may induce a decreased sense of body ownership and abnormal perceptions, such as numbness [51, 52].

Regarding alterations in body awareness in patients with PSI, it has been reported that SOA reduction is likely to induce involuntary movements [53], impair motor conversion [54], and reduce motivation and performance [55] during congruent movements. In PSI, the inputted sensory information is attenuated, resulting in, for example, inattention or indifference to the affected hand. Working to reorganize body awareness through neurorehabilitation may lead to active use of the affected hand and build a foundation for conscious and active movement in daily life.

5. Rehabilitation for PSI

5.1 Standard rehabilitation approach to PSI

Goal-oriented sensory input training after stroke hemiplegia [56] includes real-time feedback approaches to electrical, visual, and auditory stimulation, and more recently, robot-aided rehabilitation.

It has long been reported that real-time electrical stimulation of finger extensor muscles in response to voluntary movements produces excitation in the contralateral M1 and S1 regions and that electrical stimulation has the potential to improve hand motor function [57]. This approach is still being utilized today, with a 2019 study [58] describing the case of a 76-year-old male patient with hemiplegia for 8 years who underwent integrated volitional control electrical stimulator (IVES) treatment of the right flexor pollicis brevis, abductor pollicis brevis, and ulnar carpal extensor muscles. Upper limb function improved in a short period. This means that even those who have reached a plateau after a stroke may experience functional recovery of the upper extremity. Such functional improvements enhance active muscle control, suggesting that hand function is unlikely to improve if passive muscle contraction stimulation does not reach the electrical threshold for muscle contraction trigger stimulation [59]. Furthermore, it has been reported that electrical stimulation is effective in patients with mild to moderate paralysis who can actively move their hands, but less effective in patients with severe paralysis who cannot move their hands [60]. Electrical stimulation also allows patients with severe sensory dysfunction of the hand to perform movements, such as grasping cylinders and holding objects, but is less effective for skillful movements such as those performed while constantly moving the fingertips [61].

For visual stimuli, there is an approach to feedback visual information called mirror therapy [62]. Mirror therapy is an approach in which a mirror image of the healthy hand is presented in a mirror to create the illusion that the affected hand is moving as desired and to create the neural basis in the brain for the expression of motor execution. Mirror therapy has been reported to improve motor function in chronic stroke patients with mild sensory impairment and mild to moderate motor impairment [63]. Neural activity activated by this approach occurs in the primary motor cortex, precuneus, and posterior cingulate cortex, and these regions form a potential neural correlative network [64]. This means that for those who have developed discrepancies between different senses, such as visual and proprioceptive, mirror therapy may contribute to output coordination between motor output and sensory input. However, it has been noted that mirror therapy is effective only when the patient believes that "the hand in the mirror (the healthy limb) is his or her actual hand (the affected limb)" [65]. One possible reason for this is that in mirror therapy, the movement of the affected limb is not the result of movement due to active motor intention for the affected limb. It has been reported that a discrepancy between active motor imagery or intention and passive sensory information can induce abnormal perceptions, such as numbness [52], which may further degrade body awareness.

For auditory stimuli, auditory feedback is real-time phonological feedback on congruent movements, which promotes plastic changes in M1 and auditory-sensorimotor circuits and facilitates motor learning. Auditory feedback also involves M1 and auditory and integrative auditory-sensorimotor circuits [66]. However, the effects of auditory feedback on the motor learning process and the combination with other modalities, such as visual and tactile feedback, have not yet been studied in detail, so intensive experimental work will be required in the future [67].

Regarding robot-aided rehabilitation, robotic devices could help automate repetitive poststroke training in a controlled manner and increase treatment compliance by introducing them to patients [68]. The use of robotic devices allows patients to actively engage and thus perform advanced repetitive motor training, which may facilitate the reorganization of cranial nerve function and improve poststroke recovery [69]. Additionally, changes in patients can be assessed in terms of kinematic parameters, e.g., position and velocity, to capture the quantitative changes in intervention effectiveness [70]. At this point, however, the actual effectiveness of robotic training after stroke is still under debate. A review of randomized controlled trials reported that patients who received robot-assisted arm training after stroke had improved arm motor function but were not more likely to have improved activities of daily living compared to patients who received standard rehabilitation therapy [71].

5.2 Proposed new rehabilitation technique for PSI

Early intervention, task-oriented training, and intensity of repetition have been identified as determinants of motor function recovery [72]. Many rehabilitation approaches have been developed for PSI of the hand, and some effectiveness has been reported in restoring gross motor control of the hand (see 5.1. Standard Rehabilitation Approaches for PSI). However, since the hand is a part where tactile information inputs are due to minute friction from the finger pad, fine muscle adjustments are made to make it possible to manipulate an object without dropping it. It is often not possible to obtain fine adjustment strength using the muscles of the hands by simply providing strong or weak electrical or auditory feedback in response to hand movements. Additionally, an object can be grasped and controlled by synchronously matching visual information with hand movements, but visual information is used initially to define the kinematic plan of the reaching movement in the external coordinate system, and then the sensory receptors are used to coordinate the hand's motor output [73]. Therefore, the reliance on visual information lacks sensory information to monitor information inside the body, resulting in excessive hand motor output and uncontrolled dynamic friction.

What is important in rehabilitation for the functional reorganization of PSI is to restructure the body's awareness, to sense body ownership without being conscious of it, and, in other words, to be able to actively work on the paralyzed limb. So how do we develop a strategy for transformative body awareness restructuring?

As we have discussed, top-down control is responsible for predictive motor control and enables skillful movements with the hands. Since this control is built by the establishment of motor learning, it is important to establish motor learning to restore hand-motor function. Motor learning is the process of constructing and memorizing a new motor program and mastering that program and it enables behavior to adapt to the environment [74]. This neural basis is formed against a background of neuroplasticity in the brain's sensorimotor system centered on M1 and S1 [75]. The establishment of this motor learning is also closely related to the establishment of FOA and JOA in SOA. Improvement of SOA has the potential to increase neural excitation in PM, M1, and the corticospinal tracts and improve hand dexterity movements.

A necessary part of motor learning to enhance SOA is to work in situations where motor intention and sensory feedback are as temporally congruent as possible [76, 77]. Furthermore, regarding the stimulation of feedback in actual training, not only is the quantity an important factor in motor learning [37] but also the quality of feedback optimized for the body's condition and the envisaged movements [6, 78, 79]; it is important to take a comprehensive view and approach to these issues. The result is top-down control without sensory feedback stimulation [80, 81].

Based on these theories, to reconstruct body awareness associated with hand movements, in addition to synchronous matching of visual information at the expense of sensory information, a compensatory function that detects the dynamic friction that occurs when the hand touches an object in real-time is needed. Therefore, Kitai et al. [82] devised and verified an approach for sensory compensation by vibrational stimuli for vibration information (deep sensations). The deep senses are excellent at detecting pressure changes and mechanical forces associated with joint movement and transmitting them to the brain. This allows for motion control [83]. We will present a study that examined whether these concepts play a role in PSI and the impact they have on the neurological function of stroke patients.

6. Sensory compensatory training with tactile discrimination feedback training

6.1 Experiment

When the brain controls the body's movement, intrinsic receptors in muscles contribute greatly to its realization. The significant contribution of proprioceptive sensation to motor control is evidenced by a study [84] that reported that patients with proprioceptive disorders are unable to move their fingers well. In particular, PSI of the hand causes loss of reflexive control of muscles using somatosensory cues, resulting in variable muscle output when grasping an object with the hand [85]. Therefore, improving this dysfunction requires an increase in the SOA generated by temporally matching the information on motor intention and sensory feedback. This enables the hand to actively touch an object based on its functional characteristics, and real-time feedback information, based on recognition and discrimination of precise changes in sensory information caused by resistance and friction at the time of touch, enables fine adjustment of muscle output. In this study, we used the Yubi-Recorder (Tech Giken Co., Ltd., Kyoto, Japan), a real-time feedback system that enables compensatory input of tactile sensory information by vibrational stimulation (deep sensation) to other body parts with preserved sensory function, and verified the effectiveness of this approach.

6.1.1 Method

6.1.1.1 Participant

The participant was a 52-year-old right-handed man who had a right putaminal hemorrhage approximately 4 years ago and a right corona radiata infarct approximately 1 year later. The left hand was numb on a level of 11 on the Numerical Rating Scale (NRS) (0: not at all, 10: extremely strongly), with 10 indicating extremely strong numbness. There was also a loss of somatosensory and warm/pain sensation in the left upper and lower extremities. Motor paralysis was Brunnstrom stage III in the left upper extremity and IV in the left fingers. In the left-handed dexterity task, the patient needed the ability to carry small objects but had difficulty controlling object manipulation due to hand ataxia. The SOA of the left hand was decreased to 2/10, and sensorimotor dysfunction of the left hand was suspected due to the patient's complaint of "not being able to feel my hand."

6.1.1.2 Experimental procedures

To evaluate the immediate effects of training with the Yubi-Recorder on PSI in the left hand, we first performed a peg task with and without the Yubi-Recorder and then analyzed neural activity by EEG immediately after the task in both conditions. Next, to evaluate the intervention effect of training with the Yubi-Recorder, exercise tasks using the Yubi-Recorder were performed five times a week for 30 minutes/session for 6 weeks, and EEG activity were compared and analyzed after the first and last training sessions. The Yubi-Recorder is a device that can measure vibration information by detecting the vibrations that occur in the skin when the hand touches an object. **Figure 5** shows an example of a person wearing the Yubi-Recorder and performing an exercise task. The Yubi-Recorder system is capable of sensing information on the

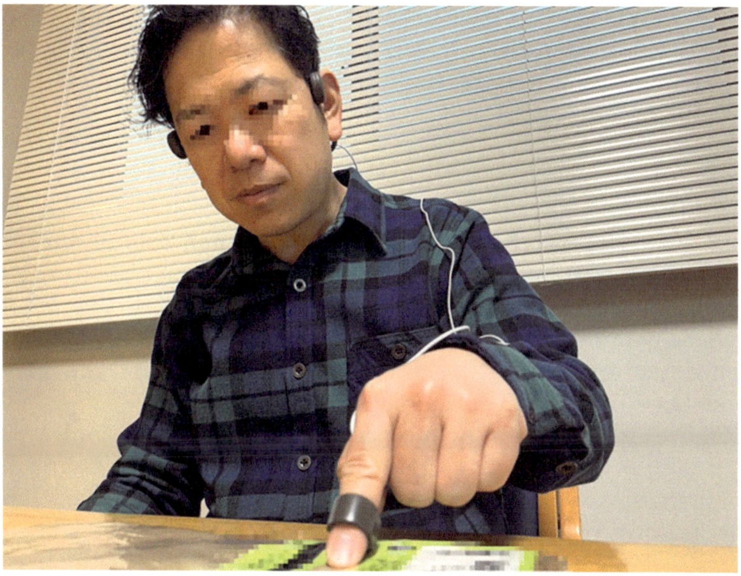

Figure 5
shows an example of a person wearing the Yubi-Recorder and performing an exercise task. A sensor attached to the left index finger senses friction information on the object, which is transmitted to a small speaker-like oscillator on the face (the mapping of the finger and face in the brain are adjacent) and fed back as compensatory deep sensory information.

unevenness, flatness, curvature, and roughness of an object and can capture tactile stimuli from any shape, thus accommodating the multidirectional motion that is characteristic of fingers. The sensor is wound around the distal interphalangeal joint of the index finger, and the output from the sensor is modulated to a frequency that is perceived by humans, enabling the presentation of vibration information via a transducer. In this study, the device was attached to the distal interphalangeal joint of the index finger, tactile information on the ventral skin of the index finger was detected as vibration by a tactile sensor, and the tactile stimulus was synchronously presented to the user's own body, through a transducer, as a vibratory stimulus. The site of attachment of the transducer was the left acromion or the left temporal bone used in the vibratory sensory examination. The method used to select the vibrator attachment was to apply five different types of sandpaper to the left acromion or left temporal bone, and the area where the roughness of the sandpaper could be identified was determined to be the area where sensory compensation could be performed. The motor tasks were to insert a steel pin with the left hand (hereafter referred to as the peg task) to stack square blocks with a base length of 3 cm used in the course cube test with the left hand and to discriminate five sandpaper pieces using the ventral part of the left index finger; each task for 10 minutes (30 minutes total).

6.1.1.3 EEG analysis

EEG measurements were derived from 15 sites in accordance with the International 10–20 method. The measured data were spatially analyzed using exact low-resolution brain electromagnetic tomography (eLORETA) analysis, a three-dimensional method of imaging neural activity in the brain. The EEG data was then calculated as brain activity values ($\mu V/mm^2$) for each task condition on each voxel in a brain region divided into 6239 voxels and expressed as Brodmann area (BA) or Montreal Neurological Institute (MNI) coordinates [86]. An eLORETA-based SnPM analysis was used to compare the Yubi-Recorder results before and after the intervention [87].

6.1.2 Results

The immediate effect was high neural activity in the non-Yubi-Recorder condition, mainly in the left orbitofrontal cortex, left dorsal anterior cingulate cortex, left dorsolateral prefrontal cortex, and left supplementary motor cortex (**Figure 6A**). In the Yubi-Recorder condition, high neural activity was observed, mainly in the bilateral primary somatosensory cortices and the bilateral superior parietal and inferior parietal lobes (angular and supramarginal gyri) (**Figure 6B**).

Regarding the effect of a 6-week intervention with the Yubi-Recorder, higher neural activity was observed in the final session compared to the first session, mainly in the areas of both primary somatosensory cortices, both superior parietal lobes, both inferior parietal lobes (angular and superior marginal gyri), and the primary motor areas (**Figure 7**). The peg test showed an improvement in the left mean from 1.5 ± 0.5 to 3.0 ± 1.0, and the learnability assessment showed an improvement in the NRS of the SOA of the left hand from 2/10 to 5/10. A motor activity log, consisting of quality of movement items, also showed improvement.

6.1.3 Discussion

In this study, in addition to synchronous matching of visual information with hand skillful movement tasks, an approach using a system device, the Yubi-Recorder, which feeds vibration information back in real time, was used to improve hand PSI. The effects of this approach were investigated.

EEG verification of immediate effects showed increased neural activity in regions of the left frontal lobe responsible for cognitive and motor functions in the Yubi-Recorder nonwearing condition. It has been shown that a compensatory increase in neural activity in the healthy motor cortex area inhibits the recovery of function in

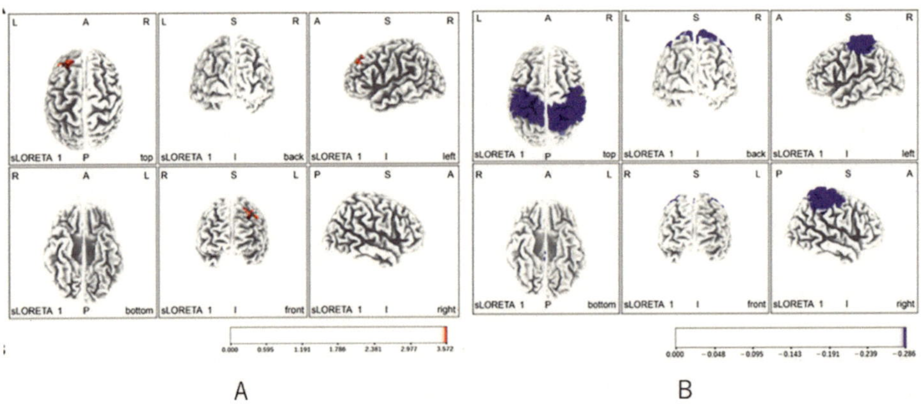

Figure 6.
Brain regions with immediate increased neural activity in the Yubi-Recorder non-attached condition (A) and attached condition (B) [85].

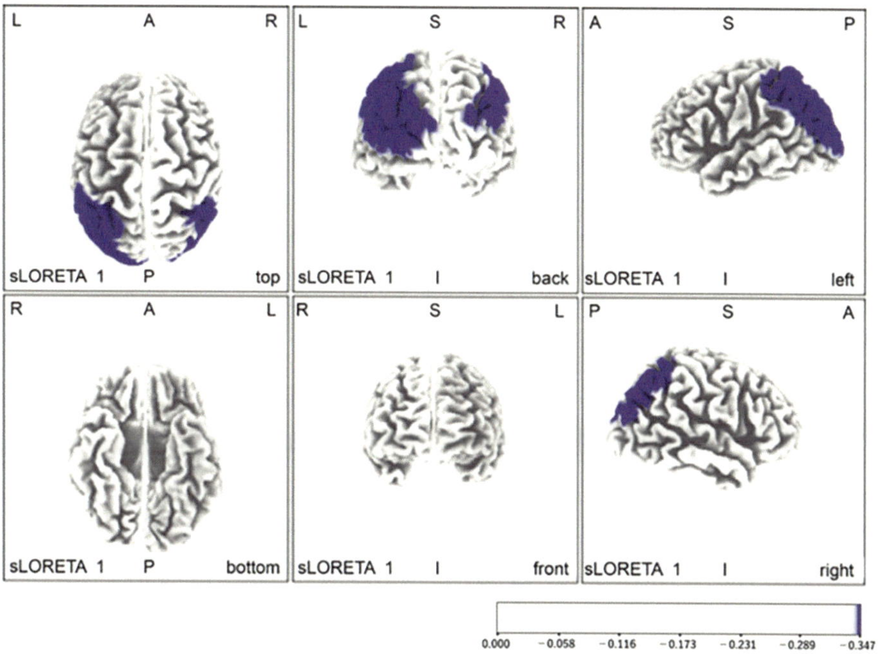

Figure 7.
Brain regions with increased neural activity after 6 weeks of Yubi-Recorder training [85].

the affected hand (interhemispheric inhibition [88]. Conversely, learned nonuse is said to progress if the patient fails to perform the intended movement even when using the affected limb [32]. The decreased SOA in this case also suggests that information collation on motor intent and sensory feedback did not match temporally and that the patient may have learned that the intended movement failed, suggesting that the left hand was not used. In contrast, the Yubi-Recorder resulted in increased neural activity in both sensorimotor cortices. Information flowing from the primary somatosensory cortex is integrated with auditory and visual information in the superior and inferior parietal lobes and stored as comprehensive cognitive information [89, 90]. The information needed for movement is then sent to the primary motor cortex, and hand-motor control is performed in the same region [91]. Thus, compensatory sensory input by the Yubi-Recorder may have immediately activated the sensorimotor areas and enhanced motor control of the left hand by making full use of these areas.

The results of the 6-week intervention were increased neural activity in the bilateral sensory and parietal association cortices and the primary motor cortex. Based on these findings, we hypothesized that 6 weeks of training with the Yubi-Recorder in this study improved peg-test performance by enabling top-down control using the sensorimotor domain during skillful movements. The motor activity log results also showed an improvement in the frequency of left-hand use and quality of movement in daily life. Motor learning is believed to produce behavioral change [92], and it is thought that the improvement in SOA in the present case also improved the frequency of left-hand use and the quality of movement in daily life.

These results indicate that training with the Yubi-Recorder can help reorganize top-down control and body awareness by cooperatively engaging the frontal lobe, where motor-related areas reside, and the parietal lobe, which is responsible for perceiving and integrating sensory information. This may serve as a rehabilitation tool for sensorimotor dysfunctions, such as PSI. This has shown the possibility of rehabilitation for sensorimotor dysfunctions, such as PSI.

7. Conclusion

Hands are an indispensable part of human daily life. In particular, to restore the most important function of the hand, "touch," it is necessary to understand that tactile perception between the hand and the object is produced by a very different principle, whether the tactile perception between the hand and the object is active or passive. In other words, we should always keep in mind that in active tactile perception, exploration takes place in the process of sensory reception, and that as stimuli, the motion command information for exploration is as important for the establishment of active tactile perception as the sensory reception information.

In the rehabilitation of hand PSI, which is the theme of this article, it is also outlined that it is of utmost importance to identify the causative mechanism of disability and implement an individually optimized approach. As an example, we showed the possibility of activating the sensorimotor domain and reorganizing body awareness by utilizing a device that provides real-time feedback on the vibrations that occur in the skin when an object is touched by a hand. We believe that the ideas described herein will be useful for therapists seeking to improve sensorimotor disorders worldwide.

This article presents several theories of brain function reorganization and motor learning in poststroke PSI patients based on neuroscientific evidence and presents an overview of effectiveness of sensory compensatory training with tactile discrimination feedback training. For this reason, it is important to understand the symptoms of PSI and the current gold-standard treatment. The development of a standardized approach is also essential to reduce treatment disparities among therapists. To extend the effectiveness of the standard approach to the fullest, it is necessary to consider appropriate feedback tailored to the patient's symptoms, such as those presented in this article.

Acknowledgements

This study was part of a research program funded by the JSPS (Grants-in-Aid for Scientific Research 22H03445). The funding source had no role in the study design/concept, data collection/analysis/interpretation, and manuscript preparation/submission.

DOI: http://dx.doi.org/10.5772/intechopen.111668

Author details

Takayuki Kodama* and Ken Kitai
Graduate School of Health Science, Kyoto Tachibana University,
Yamashina-ku, Kyoto, Japan

*Address all correspondence to: Kodama-t@tachibana-u.ac.jp

References

[1] Ikebe T, Ozawa H, Lida M, Shimamoto T, Handa K, Komachi Y. Long-term prognosis after stroke: A community-based study in Japan. Journal of Epidemiology. 2001;**11**(1):8-15. DOI: 10.2188/jea.11.8

[2] Kanzler CM, Schwarz A, Held JPO, Luft AR, Gassert R, Lambercy O. Technology-aided assessment of functionally relevant sensorimotor impairments in arm and hand of post-stroke individuals. Journal of Neuroengineering and Rehabilitation. 2020;**17**(1):128. DOI: 10.1186/s12984-020-00748-5

[3] Meyer S, De Bruyn N, Krumlinde-Sundholm L, Peeters A, Feys H, Thijs V, et al. Associations between sensorimotor impairments in the upper limb at 1 week and 6 months after stroke. Journal of Neurologic Physical Therapy. 2016;**40**(3):186-195. DOI: 10.1097/NPT.0000000000000138

[4] Meyer S, Karttunen AH, Thijs V, Feys H, Verheyden G. How do somatosensory deficits in the arm and hand relate to upper limb impairment, activity, and participation problems after stroke? A systematic review. Physical Therapy. 2014;**94**(9):1220-1231. DOI: 10.2522/ptj.20130271

[5] Coscia M, Wessel MJ, Chaudary U, Millán JDR, Micera S, Guggisberg A, et al. Neurotechnology-aided interventions for upper limb motor rehabilitation in severe chronic stroke. Brain. 2019;**142**(8):2182-2197. DOI: 10.1093/brain/awz181

[6] Kodama T, Katayama O, Nakano H, Ueda T, Murata S. Treatment of medial medullary infarction using a novel inems training: A case report and literature review. Clinical EEG and Neuroscience. 2019;**50**(6):429-435. DOI: 10.1177/1550059419840246

[7] David N, Newen A, Vogeley K. The "sense of agency" and its underlying cognitive and neural mechanisms. Consciousness and Cognition. 2008;**17**(2):523-534. DOI: 10.1016/j.concog.2008.03.004

[8] Buchholz VN, David N, Sengelmann M, Engel AK. Belief of agency changes dynamics in sensorimotor networks. Scientific Reports. 2019;**9**(1):1995. DOI: 10.1038/s41598-018-37912-w

[9] Kuriakose D, Xiao Z. Pathophysiology and treatment of stroke: Present status and future perspectives. International Journal of Molecular Sciences. 2020;**21**(20):7609. DOI: 10.3390/ijms21207609

[10] Boehme AK, Esenwa C, Elkind MS. Stroke risk factors, genetics, and prevention. Circulation Research. 2017;**120**(3):472-495. DOI: 10.1161/CIRCRESAHA.116.308398

[11] GBD 2016 Stroke Collaborators. Global, regional, and national burden of stroke, 1990-2016: A systematic analysis for the Global Burden of Disease Study 2016. Lancet Neurol. 2019;**18**(5):439-458. DOI: 10.1016/S1474-4422(19)30034-1

[12] Zancan A, Rodigari A, Gigli Berzolari F, Borrelli P. Risk factors for long-term care after hemiplegia from cancer-related brain surgery: A pilot study for new prediction model. European Journal of Physical and Rehabilitation Medicine.

2019;**55**(6):735-742. DOI: 10.23736/S1973-9087.19.05840-4

[13] Doyle S, Bennett S, Fasoli SE, McKenna KT. Interventions for sensory impairment in the upper limb after stroke. Cochrane Database of Systematic Reviews. 2010;**2010**(6):CD006331. DOI: 10.1002/14651858.CD006331.pub2

[14] Villepinte C, Catella E, Martin M, Hidalgo S, Téchené S, Lebely C, et al. Validation of French upper limb Erasmus modified Nottingham Sensory Assessment in stroke. Annals of Physical and Rehabilitation Medicine. 2019;**62**(1):35-42. DOI: 10.1016/j.rehab.2018.03.004

[15] Hossain D, Scott SH, Cluff T, Dukelow SP. The use of machine learning and deep learning techniques to assess proprioceptive impairments of the upper limb after stroke. Journal of Neuroengineering and Rehabilitation. 2023;**20**(1):15. DOI: 10.1186/s12984-023-01140-9

[16] van Stralen HE, van Zandvoort MJ, Dijkerman HC. The role of self-touch in somatosensory and body representation disorders after stroke. Philosophical Transactions of the Royal Society of London. Series B, Biological Sciences. 2011;**366**(1581):3142-3152. DOI: 10.1098/rstb.2011.0163

[17] Miyawaki Y, Otani T, Morioka S. Dynamic relationship between sense of agency and post-stroke sensorimotor deficits: A longitudinal case study. Brain Sciences. 2020;**10**(5):294. DOI: 10.3390/brainsci10050294

[18] Cramer SC, Sur M, Dobkin BH, O'Brien C, Sanger TD, Trojanowski JQ, et al. Harnessing neuroplasticity for clinical applications. Brain. 2011;**134**(6):1591-1609. DOI: 10.1093/brain/awr039

[19] Fujii Y, Nakada T. Cortical reorganization in patients with subcortical hemiparesis: Neural mechanisms of functional recovery and prognostic implication. Journal of Neurosurgery. 2003;**98**(1):64-73. DOI: 10.3171/jns.2003.98.1.0064

[20] Ward NS, Brown MM, Thompson AJ, Frackowiak RS. Neural correlates of outcome after stroke: A cross-sectional fMRI study. Brain. 2003;**126**(Pt6):1430-1448. DOI: 10.1093/brain/awg145

[21] Perruchoud D, Murray MM, Lefebvre J, Ionta S. Focal dystonia and the sensory-motor integrative loop for enacting (SMILE). Frontiers in Human Neuroscience. 2014;**8**:458. DOI: 10.3389/fnhum.2014.00458

[22] Winges SA. Somatosensory feedback refines the perception of hand shape with respect to external constraints. Neuroscience. 2015;**293**:1-11. DOI: 10.1016/j.neuroscience.2015.02.047

[23] Borich MR, Brodie SM, Gray WA, Ionta S, Boyd LA. Understanding the role of the primary somatosensory cortex: Opportunities for rehabilitation. Neuropsychologia. 2015;**79**(Pt B):246-255. DOI: 10.1016/j.neuropsychologia.2015.07.007

[24] Suda M, Kawakami M, Okuyama K, Ishii R, Oshima O, Hijikata N, et al. Validity and reliability of the semmes-weinstein monofilament test and the thumb localizing test in patients with stroke. Frontiers in Neurology. 2021;**11**:625917. DOI: 10.3389/fneur.2020.625917

[25] Johansson RS, Flanagan JR. Coding and use of tactile signals from the fingertips in object manipulation tasks. Nature Reviews. Neuroscience. 2009;**10**(5):345-359. DOI: 10.1038/nrn2621

[26] Ryan CP, Bettelani GC, Ciotti S, Parise C, Moscatelli A, Bianchi M. The interaction between motion and texture in the sense of touch. Journal of Neurophysiology. 2021;**126**(4):1375-1390. DOI: 10.1152/jn.00583.2020

[27] Johansson RS, Landström U, Lundström R. Responses of mechanoreceptive afferent units in the glabrous skin of the human hand to sinusoidal skin displacements. Brain Research. 1982;**244**(1):17-25. DOI: 10.1016/0006-8993(82)90899-x

[28] Westling G, Johansson RS. Responses in glabrous skin mechanoreceptors during precision grip in humans. Experimental Brain Research. 1987;**66**(1):128-140. DOI: 10.1007/BF00236209

[29] Knibestöl M. Stimulus-response functions of slowly adapting mechanoreceptors in the human glabrous skin area. The Journal of Physiology. 1975;**245**(1):63-80. DOI: 10.1113/jphysiol.1975.sp010835

[30] Yoshioka T, Craig JC, Beck GC, Hsiao SS. Perceptual constancy of texture roughness in the tactile system. The Journal of Neuroscience. 2011;**31**(48):17603-17611. DOI: 10.1523/JNEUROSCI.3907-11.2011

[31] Maeno T, Kawai T, Kobayashi K. Analysis and design of a tactile sensor detecting strain distribution inside an elastic finger. In: Proceedings. 1998 IEEE/RSJ International Conference on Intelligent Robots and Systems. Innovations in Theory, Practice and Applications (Cat. No.98CH36190). Vol. 3. Victoria, BC, Canada: IEEE; 1998. pp. 1658-1663. DOI: 10.1109/IROS.1998.724836

[32] Taub E, Uswatte G, Mark VW, Morris DM. The learned nonuse phenomenon: Implications for rehabilitation. Europa Medicophysica. 2006;**42**(3):241-256

[33] de Azevedo JA, Barbosa FDS, Seixas VM, da Silva Scipioni KRD, Sampaio PYS, da Cruz DMC, et al. Effects of constraint-induced movement therapy on activity and participation after a stroke: Systematic review and meta-analysis. Frontiers in Human Neuroscience. 2022;**16**:987061. DOI: 10.3389/fnhum.2022.987061

[34] Connell LA, McMahon NE, Adams N. Stroke survivors' experiences of somatosensory impairment after stroke: An interpretative phenomenological analysis. Physiotherapy. 2014;**100**(2):150-155. DOI: 10.1016/j.physio.2013.09.003

[35] Carey LM, Matyas TA, Baum C. Effects of somatosensory impairment on participation after stroke. The American Journal of Occupational Therapy. 2018;**72**(3):7203205100p1-7203205100p10. DOI: 10.5014/ajot.2018.025114

[36] Wu X, Wang R, Wu Q, Liao C, Zhang J, Jiao H, et al. The effects of combined high-frequency repetitive transcranial magnetic stimulation and cervical nerve root magnetic stimulation on upper extremity motor recovery following stroke. Frontiers in Neuroscience. 2023;**17**:1100464. DOI: 10.3389/fnins.2023.1100464

[37] Bolognini N, Russo C, Edwards DJ. The sensory side of post-stroke motor rehabilitation. Restorative Neurology and Neuroscience. 2016;**34**(4):571-586. DOI: 10.3233/RNN-150606

[38] Kalra L. Stroke rehabilitation 2009: Old chestnuts and new insights. Stroke. 2010;**41**(2):e88-e90. DOI: 10.1161/STROKEAHA.109.572297

[39] Fuehrer E, Voudouris D, Lezkan A, Drewing K, Fiehler K. Tactile suppression

stems from specific sensorimotor predictions. Proceedings of the National Academy of Sciences of the United States of America. 2022;**119**(20):e2118445119. DOI: 10.1073/pnas.2118445119

[40] Kodama T, Nakano H, Katayama O, Murata S. The association between brain activity and motor imagery during motor illusion induction by vibratory stimulation. Restorative Neurology and Neuroscience. 2017;**35**(6):683-692. DOI: 10.3233/RNN-170771

[41] Gallagher II. Philosophical conceptions of the self: implications for cognitive science. Trends in Cognitive Sciences. 2000;**4**(1):14-21. DOI: 10.1016/s1364-6613(99)01417-5

[42] Botvinick M, Cohen J. Rubber hands 'feel' touch that eyes see. Nature. 1998;**391**(6669):756. DOI: 10.1038/35784

[43] Abdulkarim Z, Ehrsson HH. No causal link between changes in hand position sense and feeling of limb ownership in the rubber hand illusion. Attention, Perception, & Psychophysics. 2016;**78**(2):707-720. DOI: 10.3758/s13414-015-1016-0

[44] Matsumiya K. Separate multisensory integration processes for ownership and localization of body parts. Scientific Reports. 2019;**9**(1):652. DOI: 10.1038/s41598-018-37375-z

[45] Schmalzl L, Kalckert A, Ragnö C, Ehrsson HH. Neural correlates of the rubber hand illusion in amputees: A report of two cases. Neurocase. 2014 Aug;**20**(4):407-420. DOI: 10.1080/13554794.2013.791861

[46] Kang SY, Im CH, Shim M, Nahab FB, Park J, Kim DW, et al. Brain networks responsible for sense of agency: An EEG study. PLoS One. 2015;**10**(8):e0135261. DOI: 10.1371/journal.pone.0135261

[47] Fukushima H, Goto Y, Maeda T, Kato M, Umeda S. Neural substrates for judgment of self-agency in ambiguous situations. PLoS One. 2013;**8**(8):e72267. DOI: 10.1371/journal.pone.0072267

[48] Sato A, Yasuda A. Illusion of sense of self-agency: Discrepancy between the predicted and actual sensory consequences of actions modulates the sense of self-agency, but not the sense of self-ownership. Cognition. 2005;**94**(3):241-255. DOI: 10.1016/j.cognition.2004.04.003

[49] Maeda T, Takahata K, Muramatsu T, Okimura T, Koreki A, Iwashita S, et al. Reduced sense of agency in chronic schizophrenia with predominant negative symptoms. Psychiatry Research. 2013;**209**(3):386-392. DOI: 10.1016/j.psychres.2013.04.017

[50] Synofzik M, Vosgerau G, Newen A. Beyond the comparator model: A multifactorial two-step account of agency. Consciousness and Cognition. 2008;**17**(1):219-239. DOI: 10.1016/j.concog.2007.03.010

[51] Miyawaki Y, Otani T, Morioka S. Impaired relationship between sense of agency and prediction error due to post-stroke sensorimotor deficits. Journal of Clinical Medicine. 2022;**11**(12):3307. DOI: 10.3390/jcm11123307

[52] Katayama O, Osumi M, Kodama T, Morioka S. Dysesthesia symptoms produced by sensorimotor incongruence in healthy volunteers: An electroencephalogram study. Journal of Pain Research. 2016;**9**:1197-1204. DOI: 10.2147/JPR.S122564

[53] Nahab FB, Kundu P, Maurer C, Shen Q, Hallett M. Impaired sense of agency in functional movement disorders: An fMRI study. PLoS One. 2017;**12**(4):e0172502. DOI: 10.1371/journal.pone.0172502

[54] Kranick SM, Moore JW, Yusuf N, Martinez VT, LaFaver K, Edwards MJ, et al. Action-effect binding is decreased in motor conversion disorder: implications for sense of agency. Movement Disorders. 2013;**28**(8):1110-1116. DOI: 10.1002/mds.25408

[55] Ziadeh H, Gulyas D, Nielsen LD, Lehmann S, Nielsen TB, Kjeldsen TKK, et al. "Mine Works Better": Examining the influence of embodiment in virtual reality on the sense of agency during a binary motor imagery task with a brain-computer interface. Frontiers in Psychology. 2021;**12**:806424. DOI: 10.3389/fpsyg.2021.806424

[56] Mazzoleni S, Duret C, Grosmaire AG, Battini E. Combining upper limb robotic rehabilitation with other therapeutic approaches after stroke: Current status, rationale, and challenges. BioMed Research International. 2017;**2017**:8905637. DOI: 10.1155/2017/8905637

[57] Han BS, Jang SH, Chang Y, Byun WM, Lim SK, Kang DS. Functional magnetic resonance image finding of cortical activation by neuromuscular electrical stimulation on wrist extensor muscles. American Journal of Physical Medicine & Rehabilitation. 2003;**82**(1):17-20. DOI: 10.1097/00002060-200301000-00003

[58] Suzuki R, Muraoka Y, Yamada S, Asano S. Integrated volitional control electrical stimulation for the paretic hand: A case report. Journal of Physical Therapy Science. 2019;**31**(10):844-849. DOI: 10.1589/jpts.31.844

[59] de Kroon JR, Ijzerman MJ, Chae J, Lankhorst GJ, Zilvold G. Relation between stimulation characteristics and clinical outcome in studies using electrical stimulation to improve motor control of the upper extremity in stroke. Journal of Rehabilitation Medicine. 2005;**37**(2):65-74. DOI: 10.1080/16501970410024190

[60] Mangold S, Schuster C, Keller T, Zimmermann-Schlatter A, Ettlin T. Motor training of upper extremity with functional electrical stimulation in early stroke rehabilitation. Neurorehabilitation and Neural Repair. 2009;**23**(2):184-190. DOI: 10.1177/1545968308324548

[61] Kita K, Otaka Y, Takeda K, Sakata S, Ushiba J, Kondo K, et al. A pilot study of sensory feedback by transcutaneous electrical nerve stimulation to improve manipulation deficit caused by severe sensory loss after stroke. Journal of Neuroengineering and Rehabilitation. 2013;**13**(10):55. DOI: 10.1186/1743-0003-10-55

[62] Ramachandran VS, Altschuler EL. The use of visual feedback, in particular mirror visual feedback, in restoring brain function. Brain. 2009;**132**(Pt 7):1693-1710. DOI: 10.1093/brain/awp135

[63] Colomer C, Noé E, Llorens R. Mirror therapy in chronic stroke survivors with severely impaired upper limb function: A randomized controlled trial. European Journal of Physical and Rehabilitation Medicine. 2016;**52**(3):271-278

[64] Nogueira NGHM, Parma JO, Leão SESA, Sales IS, Macedo LC, Galvão ACDR, et al. Mirror therapy in upper limb motor recovery and activities of daily living, and its neural correlates in stroke individuals: A systematic review and meta-analysis. Brain Research Bulletin. 2021;**177**:217-238. DOI: 10.1016/j.brainresbull.2021.10.003

[65] Franz EA, Fu Y, Moore M, Winter T, Mayne T, Debnath R, et al. Fooling the brain by mirroring the hand: Brain

correlates of the perceptual capture of limb ownership. Restorative Neurology and Neuroscience. 2016;**34**(5):721-732. DOI: 10.3233/RNN-150622

[66] Bangert M, Peschel T, Schlaug G, Rotte M, Drescher D, Hinrichs H, et al. Shared networks for auditory and motor processing in professional pianists: evidence from fMRI conjunction. NeuroImage. 2006;**30**(3):917-926. DOI: 10.1016/j.neuroimage.2005.10.044

[67] Rosati G, Rodà A, Avanzini F, Masiero S. On the role of auditory feedback in robot-assisted movement training after stroke: Review of the literature. Computational Intelligence and Neuroscience. 2013;**2013**:586138. DOI: 10.1155/2013/586138

[68] Kwakkel G, Kollen BJ, Krebs HI. Effects of robot-assisted therapy on upper limb recovery after stroke: A systematic review. Neurorehabilitation and Neural Repair. 2008;**22**(2):111-121. DOI: 10.1177/1545968307305457

[69] Liepert J, Bauder H, Wolfgang HR, Miltner WH, Taub E, Weiller C. Treatment-induced cortical reorganization after stroke in humans. Stroke. 2000;**31**(6):1210-1216. DOI: 10.1161/01.str.31.6.1210

[70] Colombo R, Pisano F, Micera S, Mazzone A, Delconte C, Carrozza MC, et al. Assessing mechanisms of recovery during robot-aided neurorehabilitation of the upper limb. Neurorehabilitation and Neural Repair. 2008;**22**(1):50-63. DOI: 10.1177/1545968307303401

[71] Mehrholz J, Platz T, Kugler J, Pohl M. Electromechanical and robot-assisted arm training for improving arm function and activities of daily living after stroke. Cochrane Database of Systematic Reviews. 2008;**4**:CD006876. DOI: 10.1002/14651858.CD006876.pub2

[72] Malouin F, Richards CL, McFadyen B, Doyon J. Nouvelles perspectives en réadaptation motrice après un accident vasculaire cérébral [New perspectives of locomotor rehabilitation after stroke]. Medical Science (Paris). 2003;**19**(10):994-998. DOI: 10.1051/medsci/20031910994

[73] Sarlegna FR, Sainburg RL. The roles of vision and proprioception in the planning of reaching movements. Advances in Experimental Medicine and Biology. 2009;**629**:317-335. DOI: 10.1007/978-0-387-77064-2_16

[74] Spampinato D, Celnik P. Multiple motor learning processes in humans: Defining their neurophysiological bases. The Neuroscientist. 2021;**27**(3):246-267. DOI: 10.1177/1073858420939552

[75] Macías M, Lopez-Virgen V, Olivares-Moreno R, Rojas-Piloni G. Corticospinal neurons from motor and somatosensory cortices exhibit different temporal activity dynamics during motor learning. Frontiers in Human Neuroscience. 2022;**16**:1043501. DOI: 10.3389/fnhum.2022.1043501

[76] Max L, Maffett DG. Feedback delays eliminate auditory-motor learning in speech production. Neuroscience Letters. 2015;**591**:25-29. DOI: 10.1016/j.neulet.2015.02.012

[77] Fourneret P, Jeannerod M. Limited conscious monitoring of motor performance in normal subjects. Neuropsychologia. 1998;**36**(11):1133-1140. DOI: 10.1016/s0028-3932(98)00006-2

[78] Koseki K, Mutsuzaki H, Yoshikawa K, Endo Y, Kanazawa A, Nakazawa R, et al. Gait training using a hip-wearable

robotic exoskeleton after total knee arthroplasty: A case report. Geriatric Orthopaedic Surgery & Rehabilitation. 2020;**11**:2151459320966483. DOI: 10.1177/2151459320966483

[79] Liu M, Ushiba J. Brain-machine Interface (BMI)-based Neurorehabilitation for Post-stroke Upper Limb Paralysis. The Keio Journal of Medicine. 2022;**71**(4):82-92. DOI: 10.2302/kjm.2022-0002-OA

[80] Patel N, Jankovic J, Hallett M. Sensory aspects of movement disorders. Lancet Neurology. 2014;**13**(1):100-112. DOI: 10.1016/S1474-4422(13)70213-8

[81] Manita S, Suzuki T, Homma C, Matsumoto T, Odagawa M, Yamada K, et al. A top-down cortical circuit for accurate sensory perception. Neuron. 2015;**86**(5):1304-1316. DOI: 10.1016/j.neuron.2015.05.006

[82] Kitai K, Odagiri M, Yamauchi R, Kodama T. Evaluation of intervention effectiveness of sensory compensatory training with tactile discrimination feedback on sensorimotor dysfunction of the hand after stroke. Brain Sciences. 2021;**11**(10):1314. DOI: 10.3390/brainsci11101314

[83] Chesler AT, Szczot M, Bharucha-Goebel D, Čeko M, Donkervoort S, Laubacher C, et al. The role of PIEZO2 in human mechanosensation. The New England Journal of Medicine. 2016;**375**(14):1355-1364. DOI: 10.1056/NEJMoa1602812

[84] Ghez C, Gordon J, Ghilardi MF: Impairments of reaching movements in patients without proprioception. II. Effects of visual information on accuracy. Journal of Neurophysiology 1995;73(1):361-372. 1 doi:10.1152/jn.1995.73.1.361

[85] Ingemanson ML, Rowe JR, Chan V, Wolbrecht ET, Reinkensmeyer DJ, Cramer SC. Somatosensory system integrity explains differences in treatment response after stroke. Neurology. 2019;**92**(10):e1098-e1108. DOI: 10.1212/WNL.0000000000007041

[86] Collins DL, Holmes CJ, Peters TK, Evans C. Automatic 3-D model-based neuroanatomical segmentation. Human Brain Mapping. 1995;**3**:190-208. DOI: doi.org/10.1002/hbm.460030304

[87] Pascual-Marqui RD. Instantaneous and lagged measurements of linear and nonlinear dependence between groups of multivariate time series: Frequency decomposition. arXiv. 2007;**0711**:1455. DOI: 10.48550/arXiv.0711.1455

[88] Takeuchi N, Izumi S. Maladaptive plasticity for motor recovery after stroke: Mechanisms and approaches. Neural Plasticity. 2012;**2012**:359728. DOI: 10.1155/2012/359728

[89] Wasaka T, Kida T, Kakigi R. Facilitation of information processing in the primary somatosensory area in the ball rotation task. Scientific Reports. 2017;**7**(1):15507. DOI: 10.1038/s41598-017-15775-x

[90] Impieri D, Zilles K, Niu M, Rapan L, Schubert N, Galletti C, et al. Receptor density pattern confirms and enhances the anatomic-functional features of the macaque superior parietal lobule areas. Brain Structure & Function. 2019;**224**(8):2733-2756. DOI: 10.1007/s00429-019-01930-9

[91] Kaneko F, Shibata E, Okawada M, Nagamine T. Region-dependent bidirectional plasticity in M1 following quadripulse transcranial magnetic stimulation in the inferior parietal cortex. Brain Stimulation.

2020;**13**(2):310-317. DOI: 10.1016/j.brs.2019.10.016

[92] Ostry DJ, Darainy M, Mattar AA, Wong J, Gribble PL. Somatosensory plasticity and motor learning. The Journal of Neuroscience. 2010;**30**(15):5384-5393. DOI: 10.1523/JNEUROSCI.4571-09.2010

Chapter 4

Intravenous Thrombolysis in Acute Ischemic Stroke

Adeolu Morawo

Abstract

Acute ischemic stroke imposes significant morbidity and mortality on patients and proves costly for the society. The most common pathophysiology involves the obstruction of a cerebral arterial vessel with a thrombus leading to distal ischemia which unrelieved proceeds to infarction. Intravenous thrombolysis has emerged as an effective and safe strategy for reperfusion and has been shown to increase the odds of a long-term favorable outcome. For more than 2 decades, the mainstay of intravenous thrombolysis has been Alteplase. More recently however, Tenecteplase is increasingly incorporated into routine practice, and it has been shown to be superior to Alteplase for recanalization in patients with large vessel occlusion, and at least non-inferior in patients without large vessel occlusion. Newer studies have expanded the time windows, introduced "the tissue clock", and included patients that were previously considered ineligible for thrombolysis, altogether increasing the pool of stroke patients with favorable outcomes.

Keywords: stroke, ischemic, thrombolysis, alteplase, tenecteplase

1. Introduction

As of 2022, stroke is the leading cause of long-term disability in adults globally and is only second to ischemic heart disease as the leading cause of death in the world [1]. Eighty seven percentage of these strokes are ischemic, while the remaining 13% are hemorrhagic [2, 3]. The toll of a stroke on an individual is enormous, but it also proves costly for society. The cost associated with stroke in the United States alone between 2017 and 2018 was about $53 billion [3]. Further, while stroke was much more commoner in the elderly, the epidemiology has continued to shift towards earlier ages with up to a quarter of strokes now occurring in people of working age [4]. Before the advent of effective reperfusion strategies, the prognosis of acute ischemic stroke was much poorer. However, over the decades, advances in intravenous thrombolysis and endovascular therapies have drastically improved the outcomes for patients with acute ischemic strokes. Even with these therapies, rapid recognition and prompt treatment are essential to optimize benefits, limit disability, and reduce therapy-related adverse events. This chapter discusses intravenous thrombolytic agents, their efficacy and safety in acute therapy for ischemic strokes, and their use in special populations.

2. Background

2.1 Causes, risk factors, and clinical presentation of ischemic stroke

Ischemic stroke is defined as "an episode of neurological dysfunction caused by focal cerebral, spinal, or retinal infarction" [5]. Non-modifiable risk factors for ischemic stroke include increasing age, prior stroke, family history of stroke, and race (Black race, Hispanic, Chinese, and Japanese) [4]. Major modifiable risk factors for stroke include hypertension, tobacco use, diabetes, dyslipidemia, a sedentary lifestyle, and poor diet [6]. Ischemic stroke presents with focal or global neurologic deficits of a wide variety depending on the locus of ischemia. The hallmark of a typical stroke symptom is its acute onset which can involve any or a combination of deficits in motor, sensory, cranial nerve, visual field, gait, balance, speech and other cognitive functions. Brainstem strokes can also cause acute impairment in the level of consciousness.

2.2 Pathophysiology of ischemic stroke and endogenous fibrinolysis

The pathophysiology of ischemic stroke involves critical hypoperfusion of cerebral tissue due to the occlusion or stenosis of the supplying artery. Common mechanisms include lipohyalinosis of small vessels; an atherosclerotic large vessel disease (via hypoperfusion through a critical stenosis, local thrombus formation and occlusion, or thrombosis with distal embolization); embolization from aortic or cardiac sources; paradoxical embolization; vasculitis from primary or secondary CNS causes; hematologic disorders; other connective tissue and inflammatory disease among others. Most of these mechanisms result in a blood clot that blocks blood flow. Blood clots are composed of cross-linked fibrin, which traps blood cells. Neurons require a constant supply of oxygen and glucose to function properly. However, their susceptibility to hypoxia and low glucose varies. Within minutes of ischemia, ATP depletion leads to dysfunction of the neuronal sodium-potassium ATPase. This causes sodium to enter the cell accompanied by water, ultimately leading to cell death and swelling. Without intervention, it's estimated that 1.9 million neurons and 14 billion synapses are lost irreparably every passing minute of stroke. This is equivalent to around 3.6 years of normal aging every hour [7].

The endogenous fibrinolytic mechanisms break cross-linked fibrin into fibrin degradation products. Circulating (and inactive) plasminogen is converted into plasmin (its active form) by the action of endogenous tissue plasminogen activator (tPA). The plasmin in turn is responsible for breaking down the cross-linked fibrin causing clot dissolution [8].

3. Thrombolysis in acute ischemic stroke

The endogenous process is limited in its speed and the scope of clot dissolution and is thus often not sufficient to prevent the rapid and permanent neuronal loss that characterizes ischemic strokes. Intravenous thrombolytic agents are designed to act more rapidly to convert circulating plasminogen into plasmin culminating in fibrinolysis. The introduction of intravenous thrombolytics (IVT) has been one of the most pivotal developments in the management of acute ischemic stroke. Several studies demonstrated that IVT use significantly improves functional outcomes in stroke patients [9–11].

3.1 Description of thrombolytic agents

Alteplase (recombinant tissue plasminogen activator or rtPA) is the recombinant form of the endogenous tissue plasminogen activator (tPA). Following the successful NINDS trial in 1995 showing improved outcomes in stroke patients, rtPA was approved by the Food and Drug Administration (FDA) for use within 3 h of onset of ischemic stroke symptoms [10, 12]. It is administered at a total dose of 0.9 mg/kg with a maximum dose of 90 mg. A dose of 0.6 mg/kg with a maximum of 60 mg is however studied and approved for use in Japan. 10% of the dose is given as a bolus while the remaining is administered as an infusion that runs for 1 h [8, 13]. Since 1996 and only until recently, rtPA has been the only intravenous thrombolytic used in acute ischemic stroke in standard clinical practice.

More recently, however, Tenecteplase (TNKase), a genetically modified form of rtPA has become studied extensively and is being used for acute stroke thrombolysis. It is an analog of rtPA with mutations at T103, N117, and K-H-R-R 296-299. TNKase is administered at a dose of 0.25 mg/kg with a maximum of 25 mg as a single bolus with the same indications, contraindications, and peri-thrombolytic care as rtPA. A higher dose of 0.4 mg/kg has been studied but found to be associated with a higher risk of symptomatic intracerebral hemorrhage [14]. TNKase has proven effective in the standard time window for rtPA and extended time windows are being studied [8].

TNKase holds many advantages over rtPA (**Table 1**). TNKase has a longer half-life of about 20 min compared to the 4 min of rtPA. This longer half-life is conferred by the former's T103 and N117 mutations. The KHRR mutations at 269–299 confer on TNKase higher fibrin specificity and 80-fold resistance to Plasminogen Activator Inhibitor- 1 (PAI-1) leading to a reduced risk of systemic coagulopathy and a longer half-life respectively. TNKase is administered as a bolus without infusion, making it easier to administer. This is particularly advantageous to hospitals that utilize the 'drip-and-ship' workflow and need to transfer their patients to more advanced stroke centers. It eliminates the logistics of managing a thrombolytic infusion during transport [8]. It also eliminates the logistics of needing an IV line dedicated to infusion. It is not uncommon to have a delay between rtPA bolus and infusion which can cause the medication to fall below its therapeutic serum level without a re-bolus. This is not a factor in TNKase use [12]. Considering all costs incurred from admission to discharge, TNKase is also less costly than rtPA [15, 16].

TNKase is superior to rtPA in patients with large vessel occlusion and the 2019 AHA stroke guidelines recommend TNKase over rtPA in these patients [17]. When administered before endovascular thrombectomy, TNKase confers greater chances of post-thrombectomy reperfusion and better functional outcomes at 3 months without an increase in the risk of symptomatic hemorrhagic transformation [18, 19]. Pre-thrombectomy reperfusion is associated with a better prognosis. Alteplase has low pre-thrombectomy recanalization rates in patients with proximal large vessel occlusions. TNKase however demonstrates higher pre-thrombectomy reperfusion rates in these patients irrespective of the time between administration of the thrombolytic and imaging assessment of reperfusion [20].

In patients with ischemic stroke who have no large vessel occlusion or who have a large vessel occlusion and are ineligible for endovascular thrombectomy, TNKase has been shown by several studies to be non-inferior to rtPA [21–23].

In a 2022 systematic review encompassing 6 randomized controlled trials and a total of 1675 patients where the use of TNKase was compared with rtPA in patients presenting 4.5 h of last known well, TNKase showed clear advantages in both efficacy

	Alteplase (rtPA)	Tenecteplase (TNKase)
Pharmacokinetics and pharmacodynamics		
Molecular structure	A recombinant form of the endogenous tissue plasminogen activator (tPA)	Genetically modified form of rtPA
Half-life	4 min	20 min
Fibrin specificity	Intermediate	High
Plasminogen Activator Inhibitor- 1 (PAI-1)	Low	Intermediate
Depletion of fibrinogen	Intermediate	Low
Dosage	0.9 mg/kg with a maximum dose of 90 mg. In Japan, 0.6 mg/kg with a maximum of 60 mg is approved for use	0.25 mg/kg with a maximum dose of 25 mg
Administration	10% of the dose as a bolus and the remainder as an infusion over 1 hour	Single bolus
Effectiveness		
Successful recanalization in patients with large vessel occlusion who undergo EVT	Poor	Much better (3-fold higher)
Favorable functional outcome in patients with large vessel occlusion who undergo EVT	Good	2-fold higher
Early neurologic improvement	Possible	Higher chances
Favorable outcome and functional improvement in patients without large vessel occlusion	Good	Non-inferior
Safety		
Symptomatic hemorrhagic transformation	Comparable	Comparable

Adapted from Zhu et al. [8].

Table 1.
Comparison between Alteplase and Tenecteplase.

and safety. TNKase use was associated with more early neurologic improvement, better functional outcomes at 90 days as measured by the modified Rankin Score (mRS), and higher reperfusion rates and better outcomes in patients with large vessel occlusion. TNKase also did not show a higher bleeding risk than rtPA [15].

3.2 Eligibility for thrombolysis

Indications for IV thrombolytic use include disabling neurologic deficits attributable to stroke (including mild disabling symptoms or improving symptoms which nonetheless remain disabling), onset of symptoms or last known well within 4.5 h of presentation, diffusion-weighted imaging positive with FLAIR-negative strokes on MRI in patients who wake up with stroke symptoms.

Contraindications include mild-nondisabling symptoms, acute or prior history of intracranial hemorrhage, history of ischemic stroke within 3 months, history of ischemic stroke within 3 months, extensive regions of frank hypodensity on CT, uncontrollable blood pressure (systolic blood pressure >185 mmHg or diastolic blood pressure >110), severe head trauma within 3 months, intracranial/intraspinal surgery within 3 months, Gastrointestinal malignancy or bleeding within 21 days, acquired and inherited bleeding diathesis, suspected infective endocarditis, aortic arch dissection, intraparenchymal intracranial neoplasm.

Specific details on the indications and contraindications as well as nuances around some contraindications can be found in the AHA 2019 stroke guidelines. It is important to note that with additional studies since the original FDA approval of rtPA, many contraindications have become nuanced context-specific [9, 17].

3.3 Time windows for thrombolysis

The initial National Institute of Neurologic Disorders (NINDS) study in 1995 proved the efficacy and safety of rtPA in improving outcomes in selected stroke patients presenting within 3 h from the last known well or time of onset [11]. Subsequently, the ECASS III study showed that there was a benefit to some patients even within the 3–4.5 h window. The study excluded patients who were older than 80 years, had diabetes mellitus and prior stroke, had NIHSS ≥25, were taking oral anticoagulants, and those with CT evidence of early ischemic changes in >1/3 of the MCA territory. These additional criteria were thus (and are still used) to exclude patients in the 3–4.5 h window in practice [9]. More recent studies however have demonstrated that these additional exclusions did not confer an increased risk of bleeding [24] and it has become routine practice to uniformly expand the traditional window to 4.5 h based on the standard inclusion and exclusion criteria only.

With advances in imaging, there is increasing recognition that the window for reversibility of ischemic cerebral tissue greatly varies in individuals, and a "tissue clock" is becoming a stronger factor in eligibility for reperfusion therapies. It is estimated that 14–20% of strokes are 'wake-up' strokes with an unknown time of onset [25, 26]. The 4.5-h timeframe thus puts most of these patients outside the window even if the stroke had occurred just before waking up from sleep. Two pivotal studies showed that using imaging surrogates to estimate an approximate time of onset or to quantify the presence of salvageable ischemic tissue can lead to a safe and effective extension of the traditional time window.

In the WAKE-UP trial, patients with an unknown time of stroke onset, but had DWI-FLAIR mismatch (focal restricted diffusion on DWI without corresponding FLAIR hyperintensity) were randomized to rtPA versus placebo. This mismatch would suggest that the onset of their stroke was approximately 4.5 h or 6 h from onset. Compared to placebo, patients given tPA demonstrated a better 90-day functional outcome without a significant increase in symptomatic intracranial hemorrhage. Notably though, patients eligible for endovascular thrombectomy were excluded [27].

Similarly, another controlled trial, the EXTEND trial, showed that patients presenting within the 4.5 to 9-h window from the last known well (9 h from the midpoint of sleep for wake-up strokes), and showing a perfusion mismatch (hypoperfusion to ischemic core volume ratio ≥ 1.2; absolute difference of ≥10 ml; and ischemic core <70 ml) had better functional outcomes with rtPA compared to placebo. There was a significantly higher rate of symptomatic intracerebral hemorrhage in the rtPA group [28]. A systematic review and meta-analyses of these studies showed an overall functional benefit in these extended time windows which persisted when the increased bleeding rate was accounted for [29].

3.4 Time dependence of efficacy

While the time window for the efficacy of intravenous thrombolytics keeps expanding, it remains true that the benefit derived remains time-dependent with better outcomes seen with earlier administration [30]. Even with a "tissue clock", the "time-is-brain" paradigm still holds. Faster administration is associated with lower odds of all-cause mortality and symptomatic intracranial hemorrhage and higher odds of long-term functional independence [31–33]. In recognition of this time-dependent benefit, institutional, regional, and national systems have been continuously optimizing their systems to achieve faster door-to-needle times while strengthening community and Emergency Medical Service systems for prompt recognition and transfer. For example, the American Heart Association (AHA) initiated the 'Target: Stroke' and has refined it over the years to provide hospitals and healthcare systems with the tools and incentives to achieve faster door-to-treatment (thrombolytic and endovascular thrombectomy) times. This initiative has been successful in achieving its objectives of faster treatment times and better outcomes [34, 35].

Mobile Stroke Units (MSU) as a system for prompt administration of IV thrombolytic have also emerged and are increasingly deployed in cities around the world. A mobile stroke unit is an ambulance with a CT scanner and trained staff who can respond rapidly to a stroke dispatch, identify stroke symptoms, perform the initial evaluation including the initial scans, and administer an IV thrombolytic on-site usually with the aid of remote consultation with a stroke provider, and triage to the appropriate stroke center [36, 37]. MSU has been shown in multiple studies to be associated with much faster thrombolytic times and better short-term and long-term functional outcomes. There is however a significant financial cost and the need to effectively integrate it into the existing locoregional system of stroke care [36, 38, 39].

4. Complications of intravenous thrombolysis

4.1 Hemorrhage

Intracerebral and systemic hemorrhage are known complications of intravenous thrombolytic use. Intracerebral hemorrhage ranges in severity from clinically insignificant to symptomatic intracerebral hemorrhage (sICH). While the NINDS definition of sICH is any hemorrhagic conversion associated with any neurologic worsening [11], the SITS-MOST definition specifies intraparenchymal hemorrhage with ≥4 points worsening in the National Institutes of Health Stroke Scale (NIHSS) score [40]. The incidence of the former is about 7% while that of the latter is about 2% [11, 40, 41]. The SITS-MOST definition is more commonly used in clinical practice as it often alters patient management [42].

Risk factors for hemorrhagic conversion include older age, higher body weight, baseline hypertension, atrial fibrillation, heart failure, kidney failure, current use of antiplatelets, extensive baseline white matter disease, high burden of baseline cerebral microbleeds, high blood pressure at presentation, higher clinical severity of stroke, extensive early changes or frank acute hypodensities on CT, acute and chronic hyperglycemia, and longer time from symptom onset to treatment [40, 43–49].

The AHA 2019 stroke guideline gives recommendations on treating thrombolytic-related sICH. If a patient develops symptoms of sICH within 24 h of IV thrombolytic use, the infusion should be stopped if still ongoing. Emergent CT head, CBC, PT/INR,

PTT, fibrinogen level, and blood group and cross-match should be obtained. The first line therapy when available is 10 units of cryoprecipitate infused over 10–30 min. If the fibrinogen level was <150, additional doses should be given. When unavailable or the use of blood products is declined, 1 g of IV tranexamic acid given over 10 minutes, or 4–5 g of IV ε-aminocaproic acid given over 1 hour followed by 1 g until bleeding stops is recommended in place of cryoprecipitate. Hematology and neurosurgical consultations as well as supportive care should run concurrently [17].

4.2 Angioneurotic edema

Orolingual angioedema is also a known complication of IV thrombolytics. The incidence of angioedema with rtPA is about 1–5% [50]. The risk is higher in stroke patients who are on Angiotensin Converting Enzyme Inhibitors (ACE-I) [51, 52]. The manifestation and severity vary from unilateral tongue or lip swelling to bilateral swelling of oral structures to rapidly progressive oropharyngeal and laryngeal edema. Most cases are however overall mild, resolving within 24 h and not requiring the need to artificially secure the airway [50]. Management of IV thrombolytic-induced angioedema involves maintaining the airway, discontinuing the thrombolytic infusion, holding ACE-I, use of IV methylprednisone 125 mg, IV diphenhydramine 50 mg, and IV ranitidine 50 mg. In refractory cases, subcutaneous or nebulized epinephrine may be required. Supportive care should be provided concurrently [17].

5. Thrombolysis in special populations

5.1 Patients with premorbid disabilities or dementia

Patients with significant premorbid disabilities or dementia have been traditionally excluded from clinical trials for reperfusion therapies in stroke. The few observational studies have also shown higher morbidity and mortality leading to pessimism and widespread exclusion of these patients from IV thrombolysis and endovascular therapies in clinical practice. However, there is increasing recognition that treatment decisions in this population is complex and must align with patients' goals while considering risks and benefits on a case-by-case basis. In the acute setting, it is better to avoid using fixed scales of premorbid disability as the cut-off for treatment or dichotomizing possible outcomes after treatment [53].

5.2 Patients with large vessel occlusion

The administration of intravenous thrombolytics (IVT) before endovascular thrombectomy (EVT) in patients with large vessel occlusion (the so-called 'Bridging Therapy') has been a subject of multiple studies. There had been conflicting results when comparing bridging Therapy (BT) with thrombectomy alone but the preponderance of the evidence, multiple metanalysis, and a real-world study are in favor of bridging therapy in improving functional outcomes [54–63]. The current American and European guidelines support bridging therapy [17, 61, 64].

There are also important logistic considerations when considering skipping intravenous thrombolysis. Most centers that manage stroke patients are not capable of performing thrombectomies and thus must transfer patients with large vessel occlusions out for this procedure. The logistics of transportation and the distance to the receiving centers often introduce significant delays in obtaining EVT. All the while, without any intervention, the ischemic core continues to expand. It is also not uncommon that on arrival and rescreening at the receiving center, patients may no longer be candidates for EVT and would have passed the window for IVT. Therefore, bridging therapy is especially important for stroke centers unable to offer EVT.

5.3 Pregnant patients

Clinical trials on thrombolysis in stroke have excluded pregnant patients limiting the available data. Indeed, pregnancy was a relative contraindication to rtPA until recently [17, 65]. Altepase does not cross the placenta and it is not teratogenic. The concern is however for hemorrhagic complications including uterine bleeding [66]. The limited case series and reports have however shown IV rtPA to be overall reasonably safe in pregnancy [66–68]. The 2019 AHA stroke guideline gives a Class IIb recommendation to consider giving IV rtPA to pregnant patients with moderate to severe strokes if the benefit outweighs the potential risk of uterine bleeding [17]. This thus calls for considering each patient on a case-by-case basis considering multiple factors and taking well into account the risk of permanent disabling neurologic deficits without intervention.

6. Conclusion

Intravenous thrombolysis is proven to be effective and safe in the treatment of acute ischemic strokes with disabling symptoms in patients meeting the criteria. While rtPA had been the mainstay of intravenous thrombolysis, TNKase is increasingly being used: TNKase is superior in patients with large vessel occlusion and at least non-inferior in patients without large vessel occlusion. Early thrombolytic administration improves the chances of excellent functional outcomes. However, the time windows for eligibility have evolved to be more inclusive with advanced imaging. Likewise, the exclusion criteria have become less restrictive and more nuanced. In special populations, such as pregnant patients and those with significant baseline disabilities, a nuanced and individualized approach balancing risks and benefits should be used in determining eligibility.

Conflict of interest

The author declares no conflict of interest.

Author details

Adeolu Morawo
Creighton University School of Medicine, Omaha, United States

*Address all correspondence to: adeolu.morawo@commonspirit.org

References

[1] World Stroke Day 2022.Available from: https://www.who.int/srilanka/news/detail/29-10-2022-world-stroke-day-2022 [Accessed: April 15, 2023]

[2] Tsao CW et al. Heart disease and stroke statistics-2022 Update: A report from the American heart association. Circulation. 2022;**145**(8):E153-E639. DOI: 10.1161/CIR.0000000000001052

[3] Stroke Facts | cdc.gov. Available from: https://www.cdc.gov/stroke/facts.htm [Accessed: April 15, 2023]

[4] Cui Q, Naikoo NA. Modifiable and non-modifiable risk factors in ischemic stroke: A meta-analysis. African Health Sciences. 2019;**19**(2):2121. DOI: 10.4314/AHS.V19I2.36

[5] Sacco RL et al. An updated definition of stroke for the 21st century: A statement for healthcare professionals from the American Heart Association/American Stroke Association. Stroke. 2013;**44**(7):2064-2089. DOI: 10.1161/STR.0b013e318296aeca

[6] Guzik A, Bushnell C. Stroke epidemiology and risk factor management. Continuum (Minneap Minn) Cerebrovascular Disease. 2017;**23**(1):15-39. DOI: 10.1212/CON.0000000000000416

[7] Saver JL. Time is brain—Quantified. Stroke. 2006;**37**(1):263-266. DOI: 10.1161/01.STR.0000196957.55928.AB

[8] Zhu A, Rajendram P, Tseng E, Coutts SB, Yu AYX. Alteplase or tenecteplase for thrombolysis in ischemic stroke: An illustrated review. Research and Practice in Thrombosis and Haemostasis. 2022;**6**(6):e12795. DOI: 10.1002/RTH2.12795

[9] Hacke W et al. Thrombolysis with alteplase 3 to 4.5 hours after acute ischemic stroke. New England Journal of Medicine. 2008;**359**(13):1317-1329. DOI: 10.1056/NEJMOA0804656/SUPPL_FILE/NEJM_HACKE_1317SA1.PDF

[10] Wardlaw JM et al. Recombinant tissue plasminogen activator for acute ischaemic stroke: An updated systematic review and meta-analysis. Lancet. 2012;**379**(9834):2364-2372. DOI: 10.1016/s0140-6736(12)60738-7

[11] National Institute of Neurological Disorders and Stroke rt-PA Stroke Study Group. Tissue plasminogen activator for acute ischemic stroke. The New England Journal of Medicine. 1995;**333**(24):1581-1587. DOI: 10.1056/NEJM199512143332401

[12] Grotta JC. Intravenous thrombolysis for acute ischemic stroke. Continuum (Minneap Minn). 2023;**29**(2):425-442. DOI: 10.1212/CON.0000000000001207

[13] A. Morawo, C. A. Adams West African Journal of Medicine 2019, Early management of acute ischaemic stroke: A clinical perspective. 36(3)286-289

[14] Kvistad CE et al. Tenecteplase versus alteplase for the management of acute ischaemic stroke in Norway (NOR-TEST 2, part A): A phase 3, randomised, open-label, blinded endpoint, non-inferiority trial. Lancet Neurology. 2022;**21**(6):511-519. DOI: 10.1016/S1474-4422(22)00124-7

[15] Potla N, Ganti L. Tenecteplase vs. alteplase for acute ischemic stroke: A systematic review. International Journal of Emergency Medicine. 2022;**15**(1):1. DOI: 10.1186/s12245-021-00399-w

[16] Warach SJ et al. Prospective observational cohort study of

tenecteplase versus alteplase in routine clinical practice. Stroke. 2022;**53**(12):3583-3593. DOI: 10.1161/STROKEAHA.122.038950

[17] Powers WJ et al. Guidelines for the early management of patients with acute ischemic stroke: 2019 Update to the 2018 guidelines for the early management of acute ischemic stroke: A guideline for healthcare professionals from the American heart association/American stroke association. Stroke. 2019;**50**(12):e344-e418. DOI: 10.1161/STR.0000000000000211

[18] Tsivgoulis G et al. Intravenous thrombolysis with tenecteplase for the treatment of acute ischemic stroke. Annals of Neurology. 2022;**92**(3):349-357. DOI: 10.1002/ana.26445

[19] Katsanos AH et al. Intravenous thrombolysis with tenecteplase in patients with large vessel occlusions: Systematic review and meta-analysis. Stroke. 2021;**52**(1):308-312. DOI: 10.1161/STROKEAHA.120.030220

[20] Yogendrakumar V et al. Tenecteplase improves reperfusion across time in large vessel stroke. Annals of Neurology. 2023;**93**(3):489-499. DOI: 10.1002/ana.26547

[21] Wang Y et al. Tenecteplase versus alteplase in acute ischaemic cerebrovascular events (TRACE-2): A phase 3, multicentre, open-label, randomised controlled, non-inferiority trial. Lancet. 2023;**401**(10377):645-654. DOI: 10.1016/S0140-6736(22)02600-9

[22] Menon BK et al. Intravenous tenecteplase compared with alteplase for acute ischaemic stroke in Canada (AcT): A pragmatic, multicentre, open-label, registry-linked, randomised, controlled, non-inferiority trial. Lancet. 2022;**400**(10347):161-169. DOI: 10.1016/S0140-6736(22)01054-6

[23] Burgos AM, Saver JL. Evidence that tenecteplase is noninferior to alteplase for acute ischemic stroke: Meta-analysis of 5 randomized trials. Stroke. 2019;**50**(8):2156-2162. DOI: 10.1161/STROKEAHA.119.025080

[24] Cronin CA, Shah N, Morovati T, Hermann LD, Sheth KN. No increased risk of symptomatic intracerebral hemorrhage after thrombolysis in patients with European Cooperative Acute Stroke Study (ECASS) exclusion criteria. Stroke. 2012;**43**(6):1684-1686. DOI: 10.1161/STROKEAHA.112.656587

[25] Mackey J et al. Population-based study of wake-up strokes. Neurology. 2011;**76**(19):1662. DOI: 10.1212/WNL.0B013E318219FB30

[26] Thomalla G, Gerloff C. Treatment concepts for wake-up stroke and stroke with unknown time of symptom onset. Stroke. 2015;**46**(9):2707-2713. DOI: 10.1161/STROKEAHA.115.009701

[27] Thomalla G et al. MRI-guided thrombolysis for stroke with unknown time of onset. New England Journal of Medicine. 2018;**379**(7):611-622. DOI: 10.1056/NEJMOA1804355/SUPPL_FILE/NEJMOA1804355_DISCLOSURES.PDF

[28] Ma H et al. Thrombolysis guided by perfusion imaging up to 9 hours after onset of stroke. The New England Journal of Medicine. 2019;**380**(19):1795-1803. DOI: 10.1056/NEJMoa1813046

[29] Campbell BCV et al. Extending thrombolysis to 4·5-9 h and wake-up stroke using perfusion imaging: A systematic review and meta-analysis of individual patient data. Lancet. 2019;**394**(10193):139-147. DOI: 10.1016/S0140-6736(19)31053-0

[30] Lees KR et al. Time to treatment with intravenous alteplase and

outcome in stroke: An updated pooled analysis of ECASS, ATLANTIS, NINDS, and EPITHET trials. Lancet. 2010;**375**(9727):1695-1703. DOI: 10.1016/S0140-6736(10)60491-6

[31] Saver JL et al. Time to treatment with intravenous tissue plasminogen activator and outcome from acute ischemic stroke. JAMA. 2013;**309**(23):2480-2488. DOI: 10.1001/jama.2013.6959

[32] Man S et al. Association between thrombolytic door-to-needle time and 1-Year mortality and readmission in patients with acute ischemic stroke. JAMA. 2020;**323**(21):2170-2184. DOI: 10.1001/jama.2020.5697

[33] Goyal M et al. Rapid alteplase administration improves functional outcomes in patients with stroke due to large vessel occlusions. Stroke. 2019;**50**(3):645-651. DOI: 10.1161/STROKEAHA.118.021840

[34] Fonarow GC et al. Door-to-needle times for tissue plasminogen activator administration and clinical outcomes in acute ischemic stroke before and after a quality improvement initiative. JAMA;**311**(16):1632-1640. DOI: 10.1001/jama.2014.3203

[35] Target: Stroke advocates the adoption of these 12 key best practice strategies for reducing door-to-needle times for intravenous alteplase in acute ischemic stroke. Phase II Phase II 12 Key Best Practice Strategies. 2017

[36] Grotta JC et al. Prospective, multicenter, controlled trial of mobile stroke units. The New England Journal of Medicine. 2021;**385**(11):971-981. DOI: 10.1056/NEJMoa2103879

[37] Fassbender K et al. Impact of mobile stroke units. Journal of Neurology, Neurosurgery, and Psychiatry. 2021;**92**(8):815-822. DOI: 10.1136/jnnp-2020-324005

[38] Turc G et al. Comparison of mobile stroke unit with usual care for acute ischemic stroke management: A systematic review and meta-analysis. JAMA Neurology. 2022;**79**(3):281-290. DOI: 10.1001/jamaneurol.2021.5321

[39] Ebinger M et al. Association between dispatch of mobile stroke units and functional outcomes among patients with acute ischemic stroke in Berlin. JAMA. 2021;**325**(5):454-466. DOI: 10.1001/jama.2020.26345

[40] Mazya M et al. Predicting the risk of symptomatic intracerebral hemorrhage in ischemic stroke treated with intravenous alteplase: Safe Implementation of Treatments in Stroke (SITS) symptomatic intracerebral hemorrhage risk score. Stroke. 2012;**43**(6):1524-1531. DOI: 10.1161/STROKEAHA.111.644815

[41] Approach to reperfusion therapy for acute ischemic stroke - UpToDate. Available from: https://www.uptodate.com/contents/approach-to-reperfusion-therapy-for-acute-ischemic-stroke#H2646531377 [Accessed: April 23, 2023]

[42] Rao NM, Levine SR, Gornbein JA, Saver JL. Defining clinically relevant cerebral hemorrhage after thrombolytic therapy for stroke: Analysis of the National Institute of Neurological Disorders and Stroke tissue-type plasminogen activator trials. Stroke. 2014;**45**(9):2728-2733. DOI: 10.1161/STROKEAHA.114.005135

[43] Whiteley WN et al. Risk of intracerebral haemorrhage with alteplase after acute ischaemic stroke: A secondary analysis of an individual patient data meta-analysis. Lancet Neurology.

2016;**15**(9):925-933. DOI: 10.1016/S1474-4422(16)30076-X

[44] Lou M et al. The HAT Score: A simple grading scale for predicting hemorrhage after thrombolysis. Neurology. 2008;**71**(18):1417-1423. DOI: 10.1212/01.wnl.0000330297.58334.dd

[45] Cucchiara B, Tanne D, Levine SR, Demchuk AM, Kasner S. A risk score to predict intracranial hemorrhage after recombinant tissue plasminogen activator for acute ischemic stroke. Journal of Stroke and Cerebrovascular Diseases. 2008;**17**(6):331-333. DOI: 10.1016/j.jstrokecerebrovasdis.2008.03.012

[46] Whiteley WN, Slot KB, Fernandes P, Sandercock P, Wardlaw J. Risk factors for intracranial hemorrhage in acute ischemic stroke patients treated with recombinant tissue plasminogen activator: A systematic review and meta-analysis of 55 studies. Stroke. 2012;**43**(11):2904-2909. DOI: 10.1161/STROKEAHA.112.665331

[47] Ahmed N et al. Association of admission blood glucose and outcome in patients treated with intravenous thrombolysis: Results from the Safe Implementation of Treatments in Stroke International Stroke Thrombolysis Register (SITS-ISTR). Archives of Neurology. 2010;**67**(9):1123-1130. DOI: 10.1001/archneurol.2010.210

[48] Masrur S et al. Association of acute and chronic hyperglycemia with acute ischemic stroke outcomes post-thrombolysis: Findings from get with the guidelines-stroke. Journal of the American Heart Association. 2015;**4**(10):e002193. DOI: 10.1161/JAHA.115.002193

[49] Tsivgoulis G et al. Risk of symptomatic intracerebral hemorrhage after intravenous thrombolysis in patients with acute ischemic stroke and high cerebral microbleed burden: A meta-analysis. JAMA Neurology. 2016;**73**(6):675-683. DOI: 10.1001/jamaneurol.2016.0292

[50] Sczepanski M, Bozyk P. Institutional incidence of severe tPA-Induced angioedema in ischemic cerebral vascular accidents. Critical Care Research and Practice. 2018;**2018**. DOI: 10.1155/2018/9360918

[51] Lekoubou A et al. Audit report and systematic review of orolingual angioedema in post-acute stroke thrombolysis. Neurological Research. 2014;**36**(7):687-694. DOI: 10.1179/1743132813Y.0000000302

[52] Hurford R et al. Incidence, predictors and clinical characteristics of orolingual angio-oedema complicating thrombolysis with tissue plasminogen activator for ischaemic stroke. Journal of Neurology, Neurosurgery, and Psychiatry. 2015;**86**(5):520-523. DOI: 10.1136/jnnp-2014-308097

[53] Ganesh A et al. Endovascular treatment and thrombolysis for acute ischemic stroke in patients with premorbid disability or dementia: A scientific statement from the American heart association/American Stroke Association. Stroke. 2022;**53**(5):e204-e217. DOI: 10.1161/STR.0000000000000406

[54] Zi W et al. Effect of endovascular treatment alone vs intravenous alteplase plus endovascular treatment on functional independence in patients with acute ischemic stroke: The DEVT randomized clinical trial. JAMA. 2021;**325**(3):234-243. DOI: 10.1001/jama.2020.23523

[55] Yang P et al. Endovascular thrombectomy with or without

intravenous alteplase in acute stroke. The New England Journal of Medicine. 2020;**382**(21):1981-1993. DOI: 10.1056/NEJMoa2001123

[56] Suzuki K et al. Effect of mechanical thrombectomy without vs with intravenous thrombolysis on functional outcome among patients with acute ischemic stroke: The SKIP randomized clinical trial. JAMA. 2021;**325**(3):244-253. DOI: 10.1001/jama.2020.23522

[57] Mitchell PJ et al. Endovascular thrombectomy versus standard bridging thrombolytic with endovascular thrombectomy within 4·5 h of stroke onset: An open-label, blinded-endpoint, randomised non-inferiority trial. Lancet. 2022;**400**(10346):116-125. DOI: 10.1016/S0140-6736(22)00564-5

[58] Fischer U et al. Thrombectomy alone versus intravenous alteplase plus thrombectomy in patients with stroke: An open-label, blinded-outcome, randomised non-inferiority trial. Lancet. 2022;**400**(10346):104-115. DOI: 10.1016/S0140-6736(22)00537-2

[59] Douarinou M et al. Impact of strategy on clinical outcome in large vessel occlusion stroke successfully reperfused: ETIS registry results. Stroke. 2022;**53**(1):e1-e4. DOI: 10.1161/STROKEAHA.121.034422

[60] LeCouffe NE et al. A randomized trial of intravenous alteplase before endovascular treatment for stroke. The New England Journal of Medicine. 2021;**385**(20):1833-1844. DOI: 10.1056/NEJMoa2107727

[61] Wang Y, Wu X, Zhu C, Mossa-Basha M, Malhotra A. Bridging thrombolysis achieved better outcomes than direct thrombectomy after large vessel occlusion: An updated meta-analysis. Stroke. 2021;**52**(1):356-365. DOI: 10.1161/STROKEAHA.120.031477

[62] Trifan G, Biller J, Testai FD. Mechanical thrombectomy vs bridging therapy for anterior circulation large vessel occlusion stroke: Systematic review and meta-analysis. Neurology. 2022;**98**(13):e1361-e1373. DOI: 10.1212/WNL.0000000000200029

[63] Smith EE et al. Outcomes after endovascular thrombectomy with or without alteplase in routine clinical practice. JAMA Neurology. 2022;**79**(8):768-776. DOI: 10.1001/jamaneurol.2022.1413

[64] Fiehler J et al. European recommendations on organisation of interventional care in acute stroke (EROICAS). International Journal of Stroke. 2016;**11**(6):701-716. DOI: 10.1177/1747493016647735

[65] Demaerschalk BM et al. Scientific rationale for the inclusion and exclusion criteria for intravenous alteplase in acute ischemic stroke: A statement for healthcare professionals from the American Heart Association/American Stroke Association. Stroke. 2016;**47**(2):581-641. DOI: 10.1161/STR.0000000000000086

[66] Demchuk AM. Yes, intravenous thrombolysis should be administered in pregnancy when other clinical and imaging factors are favorable. Stroke. 2013;**44**(3):864-865. DOI: 10.1161/STROKEAHA.111.000134

[67] Li Y, Margraf J, Kluck B, et al. Thrombolityc therapy for ischemic stroke secondary to paradoxical embolism in pregnancy: A case report and literature review. The Neurologist. 2012;**18**:44-48

[68] Tassi R et al. Systemic thrombolysis for stroke in pregnancy. American Journal of Emergency Medicine. 2013;**31**(2):448.e1-448.e3. DOI: 10.1016/j.ajem.2012.05.040

Chapter 5

Cerebral Veins and Dural Sinuses Thrombosis: State-of-the-Art Diagnosis

Dragos Catalin Jianu, Silviana Nina Jianu, Nicoleta Iacob, Traian Flavius Dan, Georgiana Munteanu, Anca Elena Gogu and Ligia Petrica

Abstract

Cerebral veins and dural sinus thrombosis (CVT) represents a rare cause of stroke. In adults, CVT has a higher frequency among cases with inherited thrombophilia, mostly women, patients with malignancy, or infections. Two pathophysiological mechanisms contribute to their clinical presentation: diminution of cerebrospinal fluid absorption and increase of venular and capillary pressure. Four major syndromes have been described as isolated or in combination: intracranial hypertension, focal neurological deficits, seizures, and encephalopathy. Non-enhanced CT (NECT) of the head is the most frequently performed imaging study in the emergency department. Features of CVT on NECT can be divided into direct signs (detection of venous clot within a venous channel) and, more frequently, indirect signs (such as cerebral edema or cerebral venous infarct). CVT diagnosis is confirmed with CT venography, which can be performed immediately after NECT, and detects the venous clot as a filling defect, or magnetic resonance imaging (MRI)/MR venography. Different imaging techniques may need to be combined to avoid pitfalls. Conclusions: CVT is a relatively rare disorder in the general population and due to its wide clinical spectrum is frequently misdiagnosed upon initial examination. The knowledge of variable clinical aspects and imaging signs will be essential in providing a timely diagnosis.

Keywords: cerebral veins and dural sinuses thrombosis (CVT), thrombophilia, headache, non-enhanced computed tomography (NECT) of the head, computed tomography (CT) venography, magnetic resonance imaging (MRI) of the head, magnetic resonance (MR) venography

1. Introduction

Cerebral veins and dural sinuses thrombosis (CVT) is a rare disease in the adult population, with a significant higher frequency among cases with inherited (genetic) thrombophilia, and young patients, especially women (due to their peculiar acquired prothrombotic conditions, such as pregnancy, puerperium, or oral contraceptive therapy) [1–5].

Unfortunately, because of its frequently misleading clinical presentation associated with the overlapping signal intensities of acute thrombosis and venous flow on conventional magnetic resonance (MR) images and MR venograms, CVT is difficult to diagnose [6–8].

CVT patients rarely appear as an arterial stroke syndrome, with an acute onset of focal neurological deficits associated with classic vascular risk factors [1–5]. Different imaging techniques are essential in precisely detecting cases with clinically suspected CVT [5–7].

Our chapter will present the cerebral veins and dural sinuses anatomy, the epidemiology, etiology, pathophysiology, and clinical and imagistic aspects of CVT [7–9].

2. Cerebral veins and dural sinus anatomy

Venous blood from the brain is drained by the cerebral veins into the intracranial dural sinuses. Familiarity with their anatomic variants or anomalies is mandatory to accurately diagnose CVT.

2.1 Cerebral veins anatomy

They consist of three groups: the cortical veins, the deep cerebral veins, and the posterior fossa veins (**Figure 1**) [3, 10]. The cerebral veins present different aspects that can determine different features of CVT: on one hand, the superficial, and the posterior fossa veins have extensive anatomic inconsistency (in number, side, and anastomoses), therefore proving why the digital substraction angiography (DSA) detection of their isolated thrombosis is problematic (with the absence of distinct cortical or posterior fossa venous territories and a misleading clinical spectrum); on the other hand, the thrombosis of the deep cerebral veins is clear to diagnose at angiography, because these

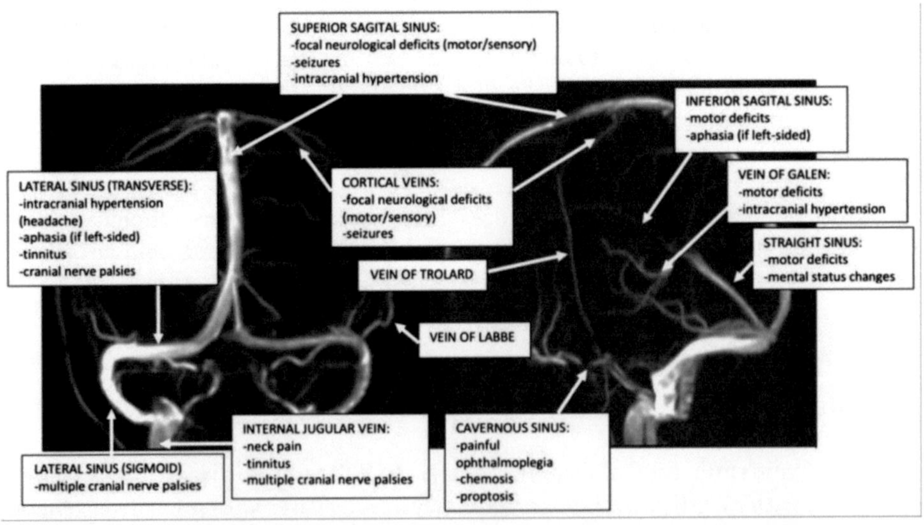

Figure 1.
Cerebral venous channels anatomy and main clinical spectrum according to the location of CVT.

veins (except for the anatomic variants of the veins of Rosenthal) are constant, always having distinct venous territories and clinical aspects, respectively [3, 10].

The cerebral veins possess thin walls and, without a muscular tunic, present no valves, with different anastomoses, which determine both their dilatation and the inversion of venous flow toward the brain if there is a thrombosis of the sinus into which they drain [3, 10].

2.2 Dural sinuses anatomy

The intracranial dural sinuses consist of a system of interconnected multiseptated endothelium-lined channels without valves, situated between the periostal and meningeal dural layers. Their walls are represented by the outer and inner fibrous leaves of the dural mater. Inside them are situated the arachnoid villi and Pacchioni's granulations, which have an important role in the cerebrospinal fluid (CSF) resorption, especially at the level of the superior sagittal sinus (SSS) and lateral sinus (LS), in which most of the CSF absorption unfolds [3, 10].

The dural sinuses are represented by two groups: the posterior-superior, and the antero-inferior (**Figure 1**).

The first group comprises the SSS, inferior sagittal sinus (ISS), LS (consisting of transverse sinus and sigmoid sinus), straight sinus (SS), and occipital sinus. The torcular Herophili is the junction of SSS, SS, transverse sinus, and occipital sinus. The second group includes the cavernous sinus, and the superior and inferior petrosal sinuses. Sometimes, the anterior portion of the SSS is narrow (hypoplasia) or with aplasia or even replaced by two frontal veins, which unite at the level of the coronal suture (explaining why its isolated lack of filling at angiography it is not enough to affirm its occlusion by the venous clot). Another variant consists of a duplication of SSS posterior portion [3, 10, 11].

Frequently (in 50–80% of the cases), the two transverse sinuses are asymmetric; usually, the right transverse sinus is larger than the left (in these cases being a direct continuation of the SSS), so an isolated lack of filling of the transverse portion of the LS is usually suggestive of hypoplasia, or aplasia of the posteromedial segment of the left transverse sinus, not of thrombosis.

The cerebral veins empty especially posteriorly, from the SSS or the SS into the LSs, and only a minority drain anteriorly, to the cavernous sinuses [3, 10].

The dural sinuses empty into the two internal jugular veins, for the horizontal position, and into the vertebral veins for the standing position. In order to avoid venous blood going back upward to the brain in cases of augmented intra-thoracic pressure, IJV present valves [12].

3. Epidemiology

Unfortunately, no epidemiologic studies of CVT contain the essential criteria for an accurate epidemiologic stroke study, due to different aspects, including the multiple nonspecific clinical features of CVT [8, 13, 14].

Current data denote that CVT is an uncommon disease, only less than 0.5–1% of all strokes [14], with a prevalence higher than previously considered, due to a raised awareness of CVT among different clinicians, and a higher accessibility to modern imaging techniques, such as MRI/MR Venography, for the assessment of ambiguous clinical aspects, such as headache and seizures [8, 13–16].

The estimated incidence of CVT ranges from 1.16 to 2.02 per 100,000 inhabitants [13]. According to different studies, CVT is more frequent in children than in adults, occurring infrequently in cases older than 65 years [8, 9]. The peak incidence in adults' population is in their third decade; thus, CVT tends to present at a younger age than those with arterial types of strokes [8]. The median age in the prospective International Study on Cerebral Vein and Dural Sinus Thrombosis (ISCVT) cohort was 37 years [7], and only 8% of the cases presented more than 65 years old [17].

CVT has prominent differential sex prevalence only in adults, being sex-independent in children and the elderly. In the 624 adult patients of ISCVT cohort, there was observed a women predominance (3:1); this imbalance is the consequence of an augmented risk of CVT in women, attributed to a sex-specific risk factor/prothrombotic condition (i.e., oral contraceptives, abortion, pregnancy, puerperium, or hormone replacement therapy) [8, 9].

4. Etiology-risk factors

There are numerous predisposing risk factors for CVT, including all factors that determine the composition of blood, especially those that can induce an alteration in the vascular endothelium or blood stasis [9].

According to ISCVT, the most frequent risk factors observed in elderly cases with CVT are thrombophilia and malignancy [17, 18].

In the Canadian pediatric ischemic stroke registry, thrombophilia was noted in 41% of all cases. Other risk factors were infections, connective tissue diseases, and neoplasms [19].

In adult patients of the ISCVT cohort, in 85% of cases, at least one risk factor was detected, and in about half of CVT cases, two or more risk factors were identified; in consequence, the detection of a first risk factor should not stop a search for possible others [9]. A prothrombotic condition was noted in one-third of all cases of the ISCVT cohort, and genetic thrombophilia was reported in 22% of all CVT cases [9]. The most frequent risk factors identified in adults with CVT are genetic thrombophilia, oral contraceptives (OC), pregnancy, puerperium, and neoplasms [9, 14].

4.1 Thrombophilia

4.1.1 Genetic (inherited) thrombophilia

In thrombophilia appears an overactivity of procoagulant factors or a deficiency in anticoagulants factors, leading to thrombus formation.

The main genetic thrombophilia as inherited procoagulant conditions for CVT are represented by: factor V Leiden (FVL) pathologic variant (activated Protein C resistance) [19–22]; G20210 A prothrombin gene pathologic variant [19, 22–24]; and hyperhomocysteinemia [25].

In a meta-analysis of case-control studies, the prevalence of FVL variant between patients' group and controls group was 12.8% versus 3.6%, and carriers of the FVL variant were more likely to develop CVT (odds ratio [OR] 3.1, 95% CI 1.8–5.5) [26]. In this meta-analysis, the authors observed that the prevalence of the G20210 A prothrombin gene pathologic variant between the patients group and the controls group was 5.2% versus 2.5%, and carriers were suggestively more likely to present the disease (OR 3.1, 95% CI 1.4–6.8) [26].

The possible connection between hyperhomocysteinemia produced by some inherited variants in methylenetetra-hydrofolate reductase (MTHFR) with CVT is still debated [20, 23, 26]. Gouveia and Canhão noted that the occurrence of the MTHFR 677C > T polymorphism in adult cases was comparable for 382 patients presenting CVT versus 1217 subjects from the control group (15.7% vs. 14.6%; OR 1.12, 95% CI 0.8–1.58). They concluded that the MTHFR 677C > T polymorphism does not represent a risk factor for CVT [27]. Marjot et al. observed in a meta-analysis, that the MTHFR 677C > T polymorphism was associated with CVT [OR 2.30, 95% CI 1.20–4.42) [20, 28]. There is no association of CVT with PAI-1 [8, 29].

The anticoagulant factors that regulate thrombin include: antithrombin, protein C, and protein S; thus, the main genetic thrombophilia as inherited anticoagulant conditions for CVT is represented by antithrombin deficiency [30], and protein C or protein S deficiencies [18, 31].

4.1.2 Acquired thrombophilia

The most frequent acquired thrombophilia observed in CVT is due to pregnancy, puerperium, OC, malignancy, and obesity [32, 33]. For example, in the ISCVT cohort of 624 adults with CVT, a sex-specific risk factor was detected in 65% of women, which represented 75% of all adult cases [9].

4.2 Pregnancy and puerperium

On one hand, in high-income countries, pregnancy and puerperium are risk factors in 5–20% of all CVT cases [9]. On the other hand, in low-income countries, puerperium is the main risk factor for CVT, with about 30% of all cases [34–37]. Usually, CVT is observed in the third trimester or in the first 3 weeks after delivery, due to the hypercoagulability state and the venous stasis that are noted during this period of time [34–37]. Pelvic phlebothrombosis may generate CVT *via* the venous plexuses of the vertebral channel, and the basilar venous plexus [34–37].

4.3 Therapy with estrogens, such as hormonal oral contraceptives (OC) or replacement therapy

According to different studies, the most frequent risk factor for CVT in younger women is represented by the use of OC [38, 39]. OC may be the single identified risk factor, or may be associated with other risk factors for CVT, such as vasculitis (especially systemic lupus erythematous or Behçet's disease), obesity [40], or inherited thrombophilia; in this last association, the risk of intra-, or extracerebral thrombosis is six times higher than that of nonusers of OC [9, 41]. A few case reports observed the association between tamoxifen (an estrogen receptor modulator) and CVT [42].

In contrast to genetic thrombophilia, pregnancy and OC are transient risk factors for CVT and they are not related to a higher risk for recurrence [34–37].

4.4 Obesity

Obesity represents a risk factor for CVT and different types of venous thromboembolism. In an observational study of 186 cases with CVT and matched controls, obesity was linked with an augmented risk of CVT for women (adjusted odds ratio

[aOR] 3.5, 95% CI 2.0–6.1) but not men (aOR 1.2, 95% CI 0.3–5.3). The risk was maximum for obese women consuming OC (aOR 29.3, 95% CI 13.5–63.6) [40].

4.5 Neoplasms

In the ISCVT cohort, malignancy was 7.4% of all CVT patients [7]. The most frequent cancers related to CVT are different solid tumors outside the Central Nervous System (CNS) (such as breast tumors or medullary carcinoma of the thyroid), hematologic neoplasms, and CNS malignancies (like medulloblastoma) [14]. The most important pathophysiological mechanisms are represented by direct tumor compression or invasion of dural sinuses, leukostasis, and hypercoagulability, which is determined by increase in acute-phase reactants, or modified coagulation factors from chemotherapy (L-asparaginase, cisplatin), or hormonal drugs [8, 14].

4.6 Hematologic disorders

Different Philadelphia-negative myeloproliferative neoplasms (MPNs) (including polycythemia Vera–PV, essential thrombocythemia, and primary myelofibrosis) develop an increased risk of venous thrombosis. However, previous studies observed that CVT is rarely associated with MPNs (especially PV). PV is a BCR:ABL1 negative, chronic MPN defined by the uncontrolled proliferation of erythroid mass due to an abnormal clone of hematopoietic stem cells, leading to an augmentation in hemoglobin and hematocrit levels and can be associated with an increase in the appearance of myeloid leukocyte cells and megakaryocytes. The Janus kinase 2 V617F (JAK2V617F) mutation led to the diagnosis of PV [17]. Other hematological disorders that can produce CVT are paroxysmal nocturnal hemoglobinuria, heparin-induced thrombocytopenia, and thrombotic thrombocytopenic purpura [14].

4.7 COVID-19 infection and COVID-19 vaccine-associated

4.7.1 CVT COVID-19 infection-associated CVT

Different cases of CVT have been reported in patients with SARS-CoV-2 infection, this type of infection being the only identified risk factor [43, 44]. According to the European Medicines Agency safety committee report concerning 34,331 cases hospitalized with SARS-CoV-2 infection, the frequency of CVT was very low 0.08% (95% CI 0.01–0.5), but with an alarming in-hospital death of 40% [45].

4.7.2 COVID-19 vaccination-associated CVT

Vaccine-induced immune-mediated thrombocytopenia (VITT) is an unusual type of thrombosis linked with thrombocytopenia, commonly determining CVT, and splanchnic vein occlusion, that has been identified subsequently to adenovirus vector vaccines against COVID-19: ChAdOx1 nCOV-19 (AstraZeneca) and Ad26.COV2-S Johnson and Johnson (Janssen/J&J) [46]. Even if there have been reported some cases of CVT subsequently to mRNA vaccines, they did not present the aspects of VITT and could have been incidental [47].

According to Perry et al. [47], when they are compared with those without VITT, cases with VITT-associated CVT were younger, had fewer associated other venous thrombosis risk factors, and were vaccinated with the ChAdOx1 vaccine. They presented extensive CVT with multiple cerebral veins and dural sinuses thrombosed, and multiple intracerebral hemorrhages. These CVT patients were more likely to present simultaneously splanchnic veins or arterial thromboses. Their outcomes at discharge were worse, with significantly higher rates of death and disability (22–47%), compared with those with other causes of CVT (3–5%) [47, 48]. The main diagnostic criteria for definite VITT-associated CVT are represented by post-vaccine CVT (4–28 days after COVID-19 vaccination), thrombocytopenia, and anti-platelet factor 4 antibodies (anti-PF4 antibodies) [47–49].

4.8 Infections

In the past, different loco-regional or systemic infections were the main etiology of CVT. Actually, in developed countries (especially due to higher accessibility to antibiotics) septic thrombosis of cerebral veins and dural sinuses (cerebral thrombophlebitis) in adults has become an unusual type of CVT (6–12%), but sometimes with significantly higher rates of death and disability [9, 32]. In developing countries, infections represent an important etiology of CVT (18% of cases) [36]. Acute infections of the middle third of the face (especially with *Staphylococcus aureus*), different paranasal sinusitis, multiple dental abscesses, otitis media, mastoiditis, or different infections of throat or scalp can determine acute cerebral thrombo-phlebitis, especially for the cavernous and lateral sinuses. Chronic CVT is produced especially by gram-negative germs or by fungi (Aspergillus). Cerebral thrombophlebitis may also develop as a complication of other loco-regional infections, such as meningitis, epidural, or brain abscesses, or after different open traumatic injury of the head, pelvic phlebothrombosis, or even after systemic infections (trichinosis, cytomegalovirus) [3].

4.9 Systemic autoimmune diseases

The most frequent are systemic lupus erythematosus (SLE), with or without the nephrotic syndrome, Behçet disease, and inflammatory bowel disease [8, 14].

4.10 Head injury and mechanical precipitants

These are rare causes of CVT.

a. Cerebral veins and dural sinuses could be occluded by different loco-regional factors, such as head trauma, brain tumors, arachnoid cysts, arteriovenous malformations, and by

b. Mechanical factors, such as neurosurgical procedures, lumbar puncture, jugular venous cannulation, epidural blood patch, or spontaneous intracranial hypotension [3, 50].

4.11 Cryptogenic (idiopathic) CVT

There is still a minority of CVT cases with no underlying etiology or risk factor. Thus, in the ISCVT cohort, no risk factors could be determined in about 13% of CVT adult cases [9], in a higher percentage for older patients (37%) [9, 17], and in a lower percentage for children (only 10%), respectively [19].

5. Pathophysiology

The pathophysiology of CVT is still incompletely known, due to multiple reasons, including different anatomic variants or anomalies of the cerebral venous channels and the paucity of experiments in animal models of CVT [9]. However, there are two pathophysiological mechanisms determined by the thrombosis of cerebral veins and dural sinuses; they are represented by the diminution of cerebrospinal fluid (CSF) absorption, and by the increase of venular and capillary pressure, respectively (**Figure 2**) [5, 51–53].

5.1 The diminution of CSF absorption in CVT cases

It is generated by the occlusion of the dural sinuses.

The normal absorption of CSF occurs in the arachnoid granulations and glymphatic system, which drains CSF into the dural sinuses, especially at the level of the SSS, LS, and internal jugular vein (IJV). In the case of dural sinuses thrombosis, a rise of the venous pressure occurs, with a consecutive decrease of CSF absorption which, secondary, elevates the intracranial pressure. This phenomenon determines an increase in venular and capillary pressure and produces vasogenic and cytotoxic edema and cerebral hemorrhage [5, 51–53].

5.2 The increase of venular and capillary pressure

It is the result of the obstruction of different dural sinuses and cerebral veins [5, 51–53].

In the initial stages of venous occlusion, a decreased but still efficient perfusion of the corresponding brain territory might be possible, due to the dilatation of cerebral veins (which present thin walls, without a muscular tunic) and, to the recruitment of efficient collateral pathways: veins of Troland and Labbe (because the cerebral veins present no valves, with the subsequent inversion of venous flow toward the brain if there is thrombosis of the sinus into which they empty). This explains why the corresponding areas of the brain can be functionally and metabolically affected, but not irreversibly anatomically damaged [5, 51–53].

As local cerebral vein pressure continues to increase, with an exceeded collateral circulation, a progression of the clot within cerebral veins tributaries will significantly decrease the cerebral perfusion pressure. Consequently, the blood-brain barrier will be affected, producing vasogenic edema, cytotoxic edema producing local venous infarcts, and venous and capillary lesions with subsequent cerebral or subarachnoid hemorrhages [5, 51–53].

The decrease of the cerebral channels drainage secondary to their thrombosis produces an increase in venous and capillary pressure, with causing vasogenic edema,

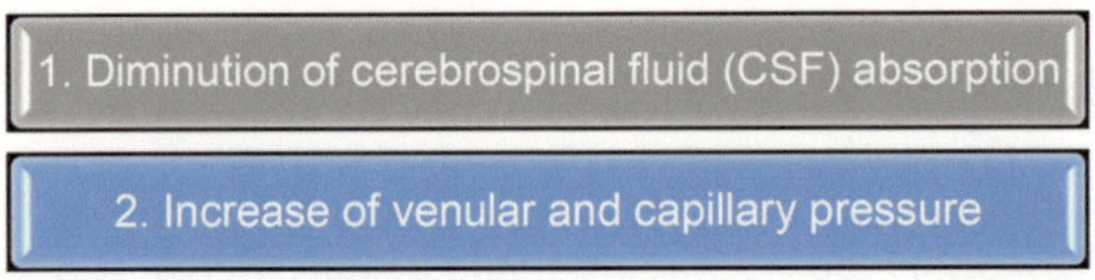

Figure 2.
Pathophysiology of cerebral veins and dural sinuses thrombosis.

with leakage of blood plasma into the interstitial space of the white matter/inside the glial cells, under the control of the hydrostatic pressure and osmotic gradients. This type of edema does not determine neuronal lesions, because the fluid in excess in the extracellular space can be evacuated [5, 51–53]. The increased intravenous pressure may lead to a decrease in cerebral perfusion pressure, resulting in diminished cerebral blood flow and consecutive failure of energy metabolism. This allows intracellular entry of ions and water across the cell membranes into neurons, from failure of the Na+/K+ ATPase pump and subsequent cytotoxic edema. In consequence, cytotoxic edema is an intracellular edema, caused by ischemia, producing the dead of neurons [5, 51–53].

Advances in understanding the pathophysiology of cerebral veins and dural sinuses occlusion have been obtained by the use of diffusion-weighted MRI and perfusion-weighted MRI, which have demonstrated the coexistence of both cytotoxic and vasogenic edema in patients with CVT [5, 51–53]. In cerebral venous infarcts, vasogenic edema is the majority in comparison with cytotoxic edema, thus explaining why cerebral venous infarcts differ from arterial ones and have a better prognosis [3, 51–53]. Brain edema and associated augmented intracranial pressure determine headache, vomiting, and diminished consciousness. In the situation of severe pressure differences, consecutive brain herniation can produce death [3].

The increase of the venous and capillary pressures determines cerebral vessel damage and erythrocyte diapedesis due to disruptions of the blood-brain barrier both resulting in cerebral hemorrhage. The neuronal lesions induced by the venous hemorrhages are usually minor than those produced by the arterial ischemic strokes [51–53].

Histological assessment in CVT patients identifies dilated brain veins, brain edema with compressed gyri, decreased sulci, small ventricles due to compression, and ischemic neuronal damages. The brain venous clot resembles different venous clot (an acute clot contains a majority of red blood cells—RBC—and fibrin and a minority of platelets; a chronic thrombus is substituted by fibrous tissue, usually with permeabilization) [3].

6. Clinical diagnosis

The clinical presentation and outcome of CVT are determined by multiple aspects, such as position and amount of occluded venous channels, the status of collateral pathways, the possible association of parenchymal lesions (cytotoxic or vasogenic edema, hemorrhage), age, gender, risk factors, and interval from clinical onset to treatment [4, 6]. Frequently, the clinical spectrum of CVT can be polymorphous, and misleading, usually with a subacute onset (in 50–80% of cases) [3, 54].

6.1 Clinical syndromes

In neonates, frequently CVT present a polymorphous clinical picture, with tetraparesis, seizures, and encephalopathy [19]. In older children, the clinical picture is similar to adults, especially with headache and paresis [55]. In elderly patients, encephalopathy is more frequent than in adults, whereas intracranial hypertension is unusual [1–4].

Usually, in adults with CVT, four clinical syndromes have been observed in combination or isolation: intracranial hypertension, focal neurological deficits, seizures, and encephalopathy [1–4]. Only a minority of adult CVT cases present distinctive clinical syndromes, such as painful ophthalmoplegia (due to cavernous sinus thrombosis), or condylar jugular syndrome-with IX-XII cranial nerves palsies (due to IJVs, or posterior fossa vein thrombosis) [1–4].

6.1.1 Intracranial hypertension

It is the most frequent clinical syndrome detected in CVT patients (40% of cases) [8], being composed of headache, associated with vomiting, papilledema, visual complaints, and sixth nerve palsy [54]. This syndrome appears usually in cases with a chronic onset [56, 57].

Headache is the most frequent symptom detected in CVT cases (about 90% of patients in the ISCVT cohort). Usually, it may appear initially isolated, and it is more frequent in females and younger adults than in males or older patients [54, 55]. Headache from CVT is polymorphic: It may be localized or diffused [56]; usually, it is severe increasing during the night and can get worse with Valsalva maneuvers or position changes (when the patient is lying down) [2, 32]. Sometimes, it resembles a migraine with aura [58], and rarely, it appears like a thunderclap headache (mimicking a subarachnoid hemorrhage) [59]. Different risk factors for CVT (meningitis, epidural or brain abscesses, meningiomas, dural arteriovenous fistulas, vasculitis) develop headache. This symptom appears more frequently in CVT cases than in patients with cerebral arterial infarcts [3, 8].

Papilledema is noted on fundoscopy in 25–40% of CVT patients, especially in those with chronic onset. It can determine transient loss of vision (usually accompanied by severe headache), and, if prolonged, optic atrophy and subsequent peripheral blindness [8, 14].

6.1.2 Focal neurological deficits

According to different studies, they are observed in 37–50% of all CVT cases and are detected at onset in 15% of CVT patients [3, 9]. Paresis, usually paraparesis, is the most common sign (in the ISCVT cohort was observed in 37% of CVT patients) [3, 9]. Additional focal neurological deficits are more rare, such as Wernicke aphasia (appears in left transverse sinus occlusion connected with a posterior left temporal cerebral venous infarct), hypoesthesia, hemianopia, and ataxia (which is noted in posterior fossa veins thrombosis) [9]. Rarely, mixed transcortical aphasia is observed in left thalamus lesions due to deep cerebral vein thrombosis [60].

6.1.3 Seizures

They can appear as focal or generalized seizures, even status epilepticus, especially during the evolution of CVT (in the ICSVT cohort in 40% of patients) [9], and less often at the onset of CVT (12–15% of cases) [61, 62]. Seizures develop more frequently in patients with CVT who present motor deficits, and with supratentorial parenchymal brain lesions, which are the result of thrombosis of the SSS and tributary cortical veins [61, 62]. A higher incidence of seizures has been noted in peripartum (76%) [62] and neonates (44%) [63]. Seizures are more frequently in CVT than in arterial strokes [61–63].

6.1.4 Encephalopathy

Subacute/chronic encephalopathy is more frequent than acute encephalopathy. This syndrome consists of impaired mental status with cognitive impairment (such as delirium, apathy, and dysexecutive syndrome), and decreased level of consciousness (varying among stupor and profound coma). Commonly, it is related with different focal neurological deficits and it is usually detected in ageing or neonate cases [17, 64]. Sometimes, the decrease in the level of consciousness is reversible; nevertheless, coma at clinical onset is the key predictor of a poor outcome [1–4].

6.2 Topographic clinical diagnosis

Because of different factors, such as frequent simultaneous multiple cerebral veins and dural sinuses thrombosis (more than two-thirds of CVT patients), different anatomic variants and anomalies of cerebral venous channels, and the status of the venous collateral circulation, the topographic clinical diagnosis of CVT is not so well-defined like in arterial infarcts [3, 9, 65]. Nevertheless, isolated occlusion of cerebral venous channels determines the following clinical characteristics (**Figure 1**).

6.2.1 Superior sagittal sinus (SSS) thrombosis

It is the commonest dural sinuses thrombosis, particularly during the puerperium (62–80% in associated occlusion and 30% in isolated thrombosis, respectively) [3, 8, 14]. Usually, it appears as an isolated intracranial hypertension syndrome. The clinical spectrum may vary depending on the simultaneous thrombosis of other cerebral venous channels, especially of the bilateral tributaries' superficial cerebral veins. In this last situation, bilateral motor/sensory signs (especially in the legs) and psychiatric symptoms (prefrontal syndrome) may be detected due to bilateral frontoparietal hemispheric lesions [3, 8, 14].

6.2.2 Lateral sinus (LS) thrombosis

LS thrombosis may develop various clinical pictures. Usually, patients with isolated LS occlusion present intracranial hypertension (pseudotumor) syndrome; less often, they accuse isolated headache. Some patients may also develop associated focal neurological deficits due to cerebral lesions determined by the progression of the LS thrombosis to tributaries' cerebral veins. Thus, fluent Wernicke aphasia appears in left transverse sinus thrombosis associated with tributaries left temporal cortical vein thrombosis (40%), frequently in association with right hemianopia or superior quadrantanopia. Right temporal lobe lesions determine only left hemianopia, without aphasia. Nystagmus and gait ataxia characterize cerebellar lesions subsequent to LS thrombosis associated with tributaries posterior fossa veins thrombosis [3, 9, 65]. Due to the fact that the left LS is sometimes hypoplastic (10–14%), the intracranial hypertension syndrome occurs especially after right LS occlusion. In such situations, a bilateral venous drainage impairment may be detected concerning the basal regions of temporal lobes and cerebellum, with corresponding temporal lobe and cerebellar signs [1–4, 65].

The infectious etiology is much more frequent in LS thrombosis than in SSS occlusion. Thus, otitis, mastoiditis, or sinusitis can produce septic LS thrombosis: "otitic hydrocephalus" [3, 65]. In this situation, the patient presents a relatively characteristic clinical picture with fever, headache, nausea and vomiting, vertigo, diplopia produced by sixth nerve palsy, neck pain, neck tenderness, and temporal and retro-orbital pain due to symptomatic trigeminal neuralgia [3, 65]. Sometimes, isolated LS thrombosis (clinically manifested with an isolated headache) could be produced by severe thrombophilia, without any associated infection (such as otitis) [5, 65, 66]. This is the reason why screening for LS thrombosis has to be performed in young females with isolated acute headache without otitis or mastoiditis [65, 66]. Rarely, LS thrombosis may produce isolated pulsating tinnitus [67].

6.2.3 Cavernous sinus thrombosis

It is rare and usually has an infection etiology, such as pyogenic infections of the face or of the paranasal sinuses [68, 69]. In cases with acute unilateral septic cavernous sinus thrombosis, they develop a peculiar clinical spectrum, with painful ophthalmoplegia, usually associated with proptosis, chemosis, conjunctival edema, papilledema, and retinas hemorrhages (due to ophthalmic superior vein thrombosis). If a fast diagnosis and an adequate treatment are missing, it progresses bilateral *via* intercavernous sinuses. When the clot extends to other venous channels, seizures and paresis may appear [68, 69]. In some situations, such as thrombophilia, surgery on intracranial or facial structures, and occlusion of dural arteriovenous fistulas, an aseptic cavernous sinus occlusion may be detected, with a poor clinical picture represented by an isolated abducens nerve palsy and mild proptosis [68].

6.2.4 Superior and inferior petrosal sinuses thrombosis

Usually, it is a sequela of cavernous or sigmoid thrombosis. The occlusion of the superior petrosal sinus clinically occurs as an isolated trigeminal palsy, while the thrombosis of the inferior one appears as an isolated abducens palsy [1–4].

6.2.5 Cortical vein thrombosis

Isolated occlusion of superficial cerebral veins is rarely detected (only 2% of all CVT cases), but it is certainly underdiagnosed, due to difficulties to identify this disease using traditional MRI sequences (spin-echo) and MR venography [70]. Occlusion is detected especially at the level of the superior superficial cerebral veins, with a clinical spectrum consisting of seizures associated with focal neurological deficits, such as motor/sensory deficits or aphasia [70].

6.2.6 Deep cerebral vein thrombosis

This type of cerebral vein thrombosis is usually associated with the occlusion of the SS; it rarely appears, more often in neonates. In such cases, its clinical picture is severe, with encephalopathy, and tetraparesis [71, 72]. In adults, a more limited occlusion of the deep cerebral veins, without associated SS thrombosis, can determine milder clinical features, especially headache, vomiting, gait ataxia, alternating hemiparesis or tetraparesis, neuropsychological symptoms, and even minor troubles of consciousness [71, 72]. Exceptional, "benign" cases of occlusion of the deep cerebral veins were reported with only mixed transcortical aphasia [60].

6.2.7 Posterior Fossa vein thrombosis

Isolated posterior fossa vein occlusion rarely occurs, because these veins possess efficient collateral pathways. However, it is the main differential diagnosis in patients with different risk factors for CVT, which present some clinical aspects (intracranial hypertension syndrome, and cerebellar-vestibular syndrome), and atypical features on brain CT, such as bilateral cerebellar infarcts or irregular cerebellar hemorrhages [73, 74].

6.2.8 Internal jugular vein (IJV) thrombosis

Usually, the IJV thrombosis appears as a progression of the sigmoid sinus thrombosis or may be determined by cannulation for long-term IJV access or can be subsequent of tonsillopharyngitis (Lemierre's syndrome). IJV occlusion can be asymptomatic, or it can manifest itself in the form of a local infection (pain and tender of the mastoid, and a painful and swelling occluded IJV). A jugular foramen syndrome (consisting of unilateral pulsatile tinnitus [67] or multiple low cranial nerve palsies VIII-XII) develops if the infection disturbs the skull base [75].

6.2.9 Emissary vein (EV) thrombosis

The emissary veins (e.g., petrosquamosal sinus (PSS)) are vestigial veins, which present no valves and link the dural sinuses with the extracranial veins. Posterior fossa EVs cross through different cranial orifices and guarantee (with the IJV) a supplementary extracranial venous empty of the posterior fossa veins. On one hand, in healthy subjects, EVs are small and asymptomatic. On the other hand, in pathological situations (such as high-flow arteriovenous malformations, IJV aplasia, or IJV, or LS occlusion) EVs become large with clinical significance (different craniofacial syndromes and pulsatile tinnitus) [67, 74].

7. Laboratory tests

Unfortunately, apart from neuroimaging, there is no simple confirmatory laboratory test that can surely exclude acute CVT.

7.1 Blood assay

According to Guidelines from the American Heart Association/American Stroke Association (AHA/ASA) a comprehensive blood count, chemistry panel, prothrombin time, and activated partial thromboplastin time are mandatory for patients with clinical suspicion of CVT [14]. The results from these tests may detect pathological processes that produce CVT, such as a hypercoagulable state, infective, or inflammatory diseases. Antiplatelet factor four (PF4) antibodies are examined for COVID 19-vaccination-associated CVT [47]. On one hand, the screening for use of OC is suggested at the first assessment of young females with clinically suspected CVT, and, on the other hand, the screening for an occult neoplasm is indicated in CVT cases older than 40 years [14, 76].

7.2 D-dimer

A high plasma D-dimer level recommends the diagnosis of CVT, but a normal plasma D dimer level does not eliminate the CVT diagnosis, especially in those situations with associated risk factors and a clinical picture compatible with CVT, such as isolated headache in young females [77, 78].

7.3 Lumbar puncture and cerebrospinal fluid (CSF) assessment

Both techniques may be suitable to eliminate meningitis in those CVT patients with isolated intracranial hypertension syndrome, and in cases with sepsis, or with fever and no clear source of infection [9, 79]. An augmented opening pressure during the assessment of CSF pressure is usually detected in CVT patients with isolated intracranial hypertension. Nevertheless, CSF assessment is not useful for cases presenting focal neurologic deficits and neuroimaging data suggestive for CVT. Unfortunately, the CSF anomalies in CVT are generic, such as lymphocytosis, hyperproteinorahia, and abundant red blood cell count, and are detected between 30 and 50% of all CVT patients [79]. Lumbar puncture is contraindicated in CVT cases with large parenchymal lesions, due to a high risk of herniation [8, 79].

7.4 Evaluation for thrombophilic state

Investigating for thrombophilia should be done for those patients who have an important possibility of severe thrombophilia (such as an individual and/or family history of systemic or cerebral venous occlusion, CVT in young adults, or in cases without a risk factor for CVT) [6]. When specified, screening should comprise factor V Leiden, prothrombin G20210A pathologic variant, homocysteine, antithrombin, protein C, protein S, lupus anticoagulant, anticardiolipin, and anti-beta2 glycoprotein-I antibodies [9, 76].

8. Neuroimaging

Neuroimaging techniques are mandatory for the diagnosis of CVT [76, 80].

8.1 Head computed tomography (CT)

Head CT is generally the initial method to be done in the emergency department in patients with acute clinical doubt for CVT [12]. It should be realized primarily without contrast enhancement (NCECT), and subsequently (if intracranial hemorrhage is not detected) with contrast enhancement (CECT) (**Table 1**) [1, 14, 76, 80].

The main advantages of head CT are: a) it may diagnose other diseases that CVT can clinically be like, such as subdural hematoma, abscess, or neoplasms; b). it may detect diseases that can themselves determine CVT, such as sinusitis, mastoiditis, abscesses, or meningiomas; c). it can identify direct and indirect signs of CVT [3, 76, 80].

8.1.1 Direct signs of CVT on head CT

They signify the direct imagining of the venous thrombus inside the occluded cerebral venous channel and can be detected in 30% of all CVT cases. They are

Direct signs	Indirect signs
• Dense triangle sign (acute clot in dural sinus on NCECT) • Replacement of normal dark flow void with a clot on MRI • Cord sign (acute thrombosed cerebral vein on NCECT) • MRI equivalent: acute thrombosed cerebral vein on T2* GRE images or T2*SW images. • Empty delta sign (chronic clot in dural sinus) on CTV/contrast enhancement-MRV	• Cerebral edema (on CT or MRI-T1 WI/T2WI) with elevated or mixed diffusion characteristics (on DWI) • Hemorrhagic infarction • Subarachnoid hemorrhage • Subdural hemorrhage

Table 1.
Computed tomography (CT) and magnetic resonance imaging (MRI) features in CVT [1].

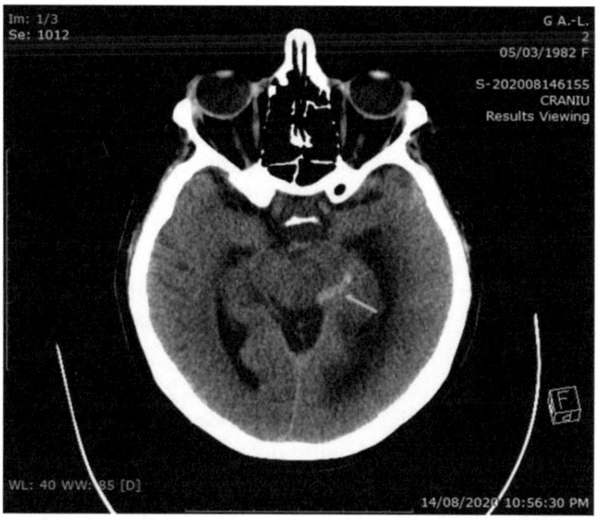

Figure 3.
Non-contrast head CT performed in the acute phase shows hyperdense appearance (acute thrombosis) of the left latero-mesencephalic vein [60].

represented by the "cord sign," the "dense triangle sign," and the "empty delta sign" [8, 76, 81, 82].

The "cord sign" characterizes an acute occluded cerebral vein on NCECT and is detected in 25% of all CVT patients. It looks as a curvilinear or linear hyperdensity determined by a fresh clot in-side a thrombosed cerebral vein (**Figure 3**) [60]. It can be detected during the first week of the disease [10]. After this period, the clot becomes isodense and then hypodense. Mimicking is detected in slow-flow patients; consequently, its specificity is considered to be rather low [3, 76, 80].

The "dense triangle sign" represents a fresh clot inside a dural sinus on NCECT, detected in only 1–2% of all CVT cases [80]. It looks as a triangular or round hyperdensity inside the sinus (usually the posterior part of the SSS) [8]. It is best imagined during the first 2 weeks from CVT clinical onset. As cases with increased hematocrit or dehydration can also determine this sign, and its specificity is low, particularly in other sinuses than SSS [81–83]. Venous sinus density quantification and Hounsfield unit-to-hematocrit (H:H) ratio have been observed to increase the sensitivity in diagnosing CVT, as attenuation of 62HU and higher is indicative of thrombosis [84].

The "empty delta sign" is observed on CECT scans in 10–20% of all CVT patients, between days 5 and 2 months after onset. It looks as a triangular hyperdensity of contrast enhancement of the walls of the sinus surrounding a hypodense central area without contrast enhancement inside the dural sinus (usually the posterior part of the SSS) [85, 86]. The sensitivity and specificity of this sign are increased to 30% of all CVT patients with CT exams with orthogonal sectioning, different window and level settings, and multi-planar reformations. Additionally, an premature separation of the SSS can be confused with this imagistic feature; consequently, it is not pathognomonic specifically characteristic for CVT [85, 86].

8.1.2 Indirect signs of CVT on head CT

These signs are more common than direct signs and are the following [9, 14]:

The intense contrast enhancement of falx and tentorium denotes stasis or hyperemia of the dura mater and appears in 1/5 of all CVT patients. The former is usually problematic to detect in chronic cases, but the latter is observed without difficulty, specifically representing SS and SSS occlusion [1–4, 85].

The cerebral veins may look dilated on the native CT assessment, due to their anatomic peculiarities (they possess thin walls, without a muscular tunic) [85]. Diffuse brain edema (20–50% of all patients) can subsequently determine an effacement of cerebral sulci and small ventricles; this latter feature may be hard to discriminate from typical aspects with small ventricles in young patients [9, 85]. The detection of the reverse sign (enlarged ventricles) cannot eliminate the CVT diagnosis, as it may be determined by the hydrocephalus due to increased CSF creation and decreased reabsorption due to increased cerebral venous pressure. Frequently, it is the hallmark of posterior fossa veins thrombosis. In both situations (small vs. enlarged ventricles), a judgment with anterior CT exams is mandatory [9, 85].

Cerebral parenchymal abnormalities may be divided into nonhemorrhagic and hemorrhagic and may be identified in 60–80% of all CVT patients [85]. The former type of abnormalities comprises extensive areas of hypodensity, produced by diffuse brain edema, as well as focal zones of hypodensity formed by loco-regional edema or cerebral venous infarction, not respecting the arterial borders. With serial imaging, some of these abnormalities may disappear ("vanishing infarcts"), and new parenchymal anomalies may be observed. The latter type of parenchyma abnormalities contains hemorrhagic infarcts, intracerebral hemorrhage, or rarely subarachnoid hemorrhage (**Figure 4**) [8, 60, 85].

Some types of CVT may develop on CT peculiar aspects.

First, numerous irregular filling defects with distended cavernous sinuses and orbital veins on CECT are mandatory for cavernous sinus thrombosis [14, 76]. Second, bilateral parasagittal hemispheric lesions are very evocative for occlusion of the SSS [14, 76]. Third, temporo-occipital lesions designate LS or vein of Labbe thrombosis [14, 76]. Fourth, in patients with acute deep cerebral veins occlusion, they present bilateral hypodensities, representing thalami, basal ganglia, and internal capsule infarcts; bilateral hyper-densities with the same location, determined by acute cerebral hemorrhages or hemorrhagic infarcts; extensive edema with compression of the third ventricle and subsequent hydrocephalus, and a hyperdense area inside the occluded sinuses, due to a fresh clot. In consequence, the presence of hemorrhage or edema adjacent to a cerebral venous channel should recommend CVT [14, 76]. Fifth, cerebellar venous infarctions can produce hydrocephalus and compression of the fourth ventricle [14, 76].

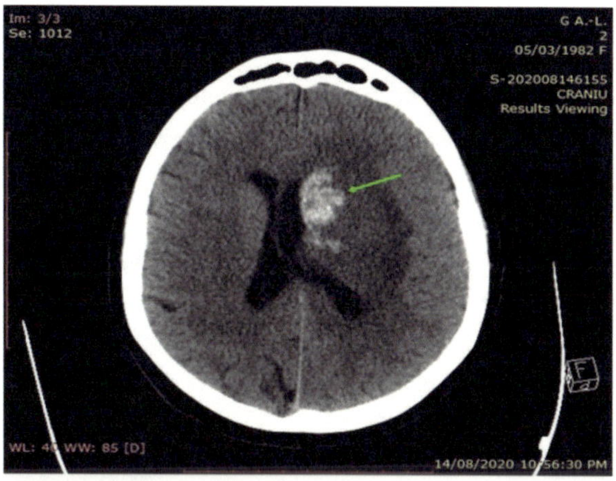

Figure 4.
Non-contrast head CT performed in the acute phase shows venous infarction with hemorrhagic transformation in corpus of the left caudate nucleus [60].

Regrettably, head CT detection of CVT is insensitive, results being pathological only in 30% of true CVT subjects, and all CT signs are nonspecific in the other patients [14]. Additionally, different anatomic variants may mimic sinus occlusion, such as sinus atresia or hypoplasia, asymmetric sinus drainage, and normal sinus filling defects related to arachnoid granulations or intrasinus septa [14, 76]. Consequently, a normal Head CT will not eliminate a CVT. So, in clinically supposed cases, a CT venography or MRI venography is mandatory for CVT detection [81, 82].

8.2 CT venography-CTV (multi-detector CT angiography-MDCTA) with bolus injection of contrast material

Usually, CT venography (CTV) is done especially in acute CVT patients, immediately after NCECT. It certifies an excellent detection of the venous channels (high-density contrast in patent segments) (**Table 2**) [1].

CTV can distinguish both direct signs of thrombosis (filling defects, with low density in the occluded venous channels) and indirect signs (sinus wall enhancement and increased collateral venous circulation). Supplementary, in subacute or chronic CVT cases, CTV can detect a heterogeneous thrombus (**Table 2**) [8, 85].

When CTV accompanies head CT, their combined accuracy is 90–100%, depending on the obstruction location [86–90].

CTV presents some advantages versus digital subtraction intra-arterial angiography (DSA): It is cheaper, less invasive, and quicker (due to a faster image acquisition). CTV identifies better the ISS, the cavernous sinuses, and the basal vein of Rosenthal (with multiplanar reformatted images) than DSA [87–90]. Compared with DSA, the combination of CT/CTV has a sensitivity and specificity of 95 and 91%, respectively [14].

CTV offers some advantages compared to magnetic resonance venography (MRV): It is much more reachable, cheaper, faster, has no contraindications to ferromagnetic devices, amplified imaging resolution for the main dural sinuses, easier to comprehend, and has fewer artifacts than MRV. CTV presents a similar accuracy as time-of-flight (TOF) MRV in the detection of the dural sinuses, with

Imaging method	Advantages	Disadvantages
CTV	• More widely accessible than MRV • Generally, costs less than MRV • Faster image acquisition than MRV • More suitable for unstable patients. • Less prone to motion artifact. • Better detection of cerebral small vessels.	• Radiation risk • Higher rate of adverse reactions to iodinated contrasts, including the risk of contrast-induced nephropathy. • Potentially reduced visualization of skull base structures in 3D display. • Acute thrombus, which is hyperdense, may mimic opacified sinus, resulting in false-negative results.
MRV	• No radiation risk • Low rate of adverse reactions to Gadolinium. • Indicated in cases with severe renal failure if done without contrast enhancement contrast technique). • Higher sensitivity for small parenchymal lesions.	• Contraindicated in cases with ferromagnetic devices and most pacemakers. • More prone to motion artifact. • TOF-MRV may present false-positive results from a flow that has a parallel direction with the acquisition plane. • For this reason, phase-contrast MRV has to be used to identify the thrombus. • Stenotic, hypoplastic, or aplastic dural sinuses may be misdiagnosed as CVT.
CTV and MRV	Noninvasive imaging methods with indirect signs possible to detect.	• Inferior resolution to detect the patency of the posterior part or entire SSS, both LSs of the deep cerebral veins to DSA.

Table 2.
Comparison of CTV and MRV in CVT [1].

higher ability versus MRV to detect: the ISS and the nondominant transverse sinus occlusion; the single cortical vein thrombosis; and venous channels with low flow [87–90]. Regrettably, CTV is less sensitive in the valuation of the superficial and deep cerebral veins than in that of the dural sinuses. This weakness can be perfected by using multiplanar reformations, which growths the sensitivity of CTV beyond DSA [87, 88]. Unfortunately, maximum intensity projection (MIP) image generation has reduced recognition of skull base components in three-dimensional display, with unintended sinus omission from bone subtracting algorithms. Nevertheless, this can be ameliorated with specific software for mask bone elimination [90]. CTV also has some disadvantages, such as contrast allergy, contrast nephropathy due to contrast material, and radiation exposure, which may contraindicate its usage during pregnancy or renal failure [90].

8.3 Magnetic resonance imaging (MRI) of the head

Unenhanced MRI is a more sensitive technique for detecting CVT than NECT. Patent dural sinuses can be seen as flow voids (hyposignal on T1, and T2 WI) on MRI [91, 92].

MRI pathological signs in CVT patients consist of direct signs (detecting the thrombus itself inside the venous channel) and indirect signs, respectively (lesions secondary to venous occlusion, perceived especially at the level of the cerebral parenchyma) [91, 92].

8.3.1 The MRI direct signs

The key signs of thrombosis are represented by the replacement of normal dark flow void (which certifies the presence of flow inside a patent venous channel) with the absence of a flow void (which denotes the absence of flow in an occluded cerebral venous channel). The signal intensity of the venous clot on T1- and T2-weighted MR images is comparable to a hematoma, and it is developing dependent on thrombus oldness. The consecutive signal intensity changes observed in the thrombus are the consequences of the paramagnetic aspects of the hemoglobin and its degradation products (i.e., hemosiderin, methemoglobin, deoxyhemoglobin) (**Table 3**) [82, 91–96].

a. In the acute phase (the first 5 days after the clinical onset), the flow void is missing (the vessel is occluded with absence of flow) and the thrombosed venous channel is isointense with brain tissue on T1-WI and hypo/isointense on T2-WI, as a result of the richness of deoxyhemoglobin in RBC inside the thrombus. The recognition of CVT (fresh venous clot) in the acute stage is problematic on single conventional MRI, because the MRI signs are comparable to normal venous flow. Therefore, other MRI sequences, MRV, CTV, or DSA are required to identify the absence of flow in the occluded cerebral veins or dural sinuses [91, 92].

b. In the subacute phase (between 6 and 15–30 days after the clinical onset), the thrombus becomes more apparent because the signal is hyperintense in both T1- and T2-WI, due to the accumulation of methemoglobin inside the clot. These imaging signs are specific for CVT and are the most common imagistic features (**Figure 5**) [89–92].

c. In the chronic stage (between 2 and 4 weeks after the clinical onset), the commencement of recanalization of the previously thrombosed venous channel produces the reappearance of the flow void (the vessel is now patent). In this stage, the venous thrombus, which is heterogeneous, is isointense on T1-WI, with variable intensity (iso/hyperintense) on T2-WI, due to the deoxygenated hemoglobin and methemoglobin components. Therefore, in this stage, the diagnosis of CVT can be unnoticed [91, 92].

After 4–6 months, no signal anomaly is observed on T1-WI or DWI; nevertheless, delicate changes (heterogeneous topic signal abnormalities) can be detected in T2-WI or FLAIR, which can persist for years, and should not be interpreted for a recurrent acute CVT [91, 92].

	Normal sinus	Thrombus less than 5 days old	Thrombus from D5 to D30	Thrombus older than 1 month
T1	Hyposignal	Isosignal	Hypersignal	Iso/hypersignal
T2	Hyposignal	Hypo/isosignal	Iso/hypersignal	Iso/hypersignal
Contrast-enhanced T1	Homogeneous because the fresh thrombus can be enhanced	Empty delta sign	Empty delta sign	Empty delta

Table 3.
The evolution of the thrombus signal [82].

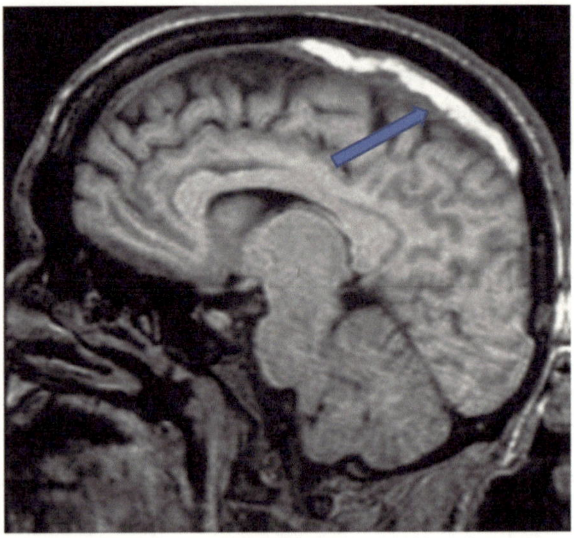

Figure 5.
MRI midline sagittal T1-weighted image. Blue arrow—hyper-intense signal indicating subacute thrombosis of the SSS; this pattern was found 14 days after the onset of symptoms.

Regrettably, in a substantial percent of cases, we can notice false-negative or false-positive appearances. The false-negative situations are infrequent and characterize a supra-acute or chronic stage, or a single superficial cerebral vein occlusion, which will be detected mainly by DSA. The false-positive conditions are the consequence of slowly cerebral venous flow. To diminish both artifacts, we have to change the position of the subject, to repeat the sequence in another plane, with two or more sequences, and with other types of sequences, as follows [76, 85]:

Gradient echo T2-weighted (T2*GRE) MRI sequences*: Recognize CVT, as degradation products, which can determine augmented signal drop-out, identifying intravenous channels thrombus in stages where the clot can be barely visible in other sequences [93]. Consequently, on T2*GRE MRI sequences, the fresh thrombus can be identified as an area of hypointensity in the affected venous channel. Nevertheless, a chronically occluded dural sinus may still present hypo signal on *T2*GRE* [94].

*Echo-planar T2 susceptibility weighted imaging (T2*SWI) MRI sequences*: It is a complementary T2* GRE sequence to assess CVT. SWI detects the acute isolated superficial cerebral veins occlusion, when both T1 and T2 are less sensitive. It identifies the intraluminal thrombus as a hypointense area. The exaggeration of magnetic susceptibility effect (MSE) aids recognition of discrete thrombosis, and supplementary, this sequence distinguishes cerebral venous stasis, existence of collateral circulation, and intracranial hemorrhage [95]. Complementary, SWI shows a blooming artifact better detected than T2* GRE, determining a better position of the clot or hemorrhage. Isolated superficial cerebral vein occlusion may be easier to diagnose on the maximum-intensity projections (MIPs) of SWI compared to dedicate venous imaging [82, 95].

8.3.2 The MRI indirect signs

Different cerebral lesions secondary to venous channel occlusion, such as brain edema, cerebral infarct, and/or cerebral hemorrhage, observed in CVT patients are better identified by MRI than by CT [81].

Cerebral edema and cerebral venous infarction determine both a hypersignal on T2-WI and an isointense/hypointense signal on T1-WI. Isolated cerebral edema, without associated cerebral venous infarcts or cerebral hemorrhages, may be detected in near half of CVT cases and may be accompanied with cortical sulcal effacement and small ventricles. When these MRI features are identified, CTV or MRV should be done to endorse the CVT diagnosis [91, 92].

Cerebral hemorrhage is characterized by a hypersignal in both T1- and T2- WI, occurring in 30% of all CVT cases. Frequently, SSS thrombosis may be associated with flame-shaped, irregular, and heterogeneous bilateral parasagittal areas of frontoparietal hemorrhages. Usually, LS occlusion is accompanied by both temporal and occipital lobes lesions. The occlusion of the vein of Galen or of the SS may be associated with bilateral deep brain lesions, such as thalamic hemorrhages, intraventricular hemorrhages, or wide brain edema [91, 92].

Unfortunately, there is no simple confirmatory MRI indirect sign for CVT, but their significance is clear because of the concomitant MRI direct signs for CVT [91, 92].

Diffusion-weighted imaging (DWI) techniques: DWI detects the thrombus as a hypersignal inside the occluded venous channel, with a reduced apparent diffusion coefficient (ADC). Patients with restriction on DWI have extended recovery time and lower probability of total clot recanalization (DWI-prognostic factor) [14, 96] (**Figure 6**).

DWI identifies cerebral edema, which may be divided in:

- Vasogenic edema, presenting diverse signal deviations in the damaged regions, and raised ADC values, lacking lesser ADC values than in health areas [1, 94].

- Cytotoxic edema, presenting a hypersignal, and low ADC values [1, 94].

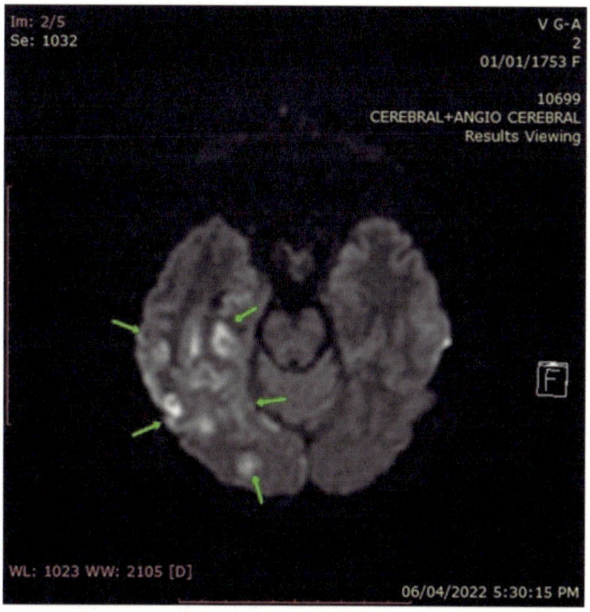

Figure 6.
DWI-b1000. Non-contrast head MRI performed in the acute phase shows a large venous infarction in right temporal lobe (arrows).

On perfusion-weighted (PWI) MRI, relative cerebral blood volume (rCBV), and mean transit time (MTT) are augmented in damaged regions, with conserved relative cerebral blood flow (rCBF) [1–4, 96].

Usually, in CVT patients, the vasogenic edema is prominent versus cytotoxic edema; in consequence, the corresponding cerebral areas may be functionally and metabolically affected, but not irreversibly. The reversibility of venous brain lesions is emblematic for CVT patients, determining both a better recovery in venous cerebral ischemic strokes than in arterial infarcts and vanishing lesions on MRI, respectively [91–96].

8.4 Magnetic resonance venography (MRV)

MRV may be realized without contrast enhancement (using TOF technique or phase-contrast technique) or with a contrast-enhanced technique [97, 98].

8.4.1 The two-dimensional (2D-TOF) technique (with 1.5- and 3-mm thick slices in the coronal and axial planes)

This technique is mandatory in pregnant or breastfeeding females, or in patients with severe renal failure, where contrast enhancement is proscribed. It detects: a). the direct sign of CVT, represented by the absence of flow signal (nonappearance of opacification) of venous channel, though interpretation can be confused by different anatomic variants, like sinus hypoplasia, or asymmetric flow [97, 98]. b). The indirect signs of CVT comprise delayed emptying, collateral venous circulation, dilated veins, and tortuous collateral cortical veins (corkscrew veins) (**Figure 7**) [4].

2D-TOF technique is superior to its 3D counterpart, because it has a relative absence of saturation effects and superior sensitivity in the setting of slow venous flow but presents a low sensitivity to small cerebral veins with slow flow. One significant pitfall is that same-plane acquisition can produce false-positive results from saturation and subsequent signal nulling, as this technique is most sensitive to orthogonal flow [97, 98].

8.4.2 Contrast-enhanced (CE)-MRV (MRV with gadolinium)

MRV with gadolinium realizes a direct examination of luminal filling similar to that of CTV, with similar sensitivity and specificity (**Figure 8**). Both CTV and CE-MRV are superior to the TOF and phase-contrast (PC) techniques, due to different artifacts that may be observed in these sequences [85]. Regrettably, conventional MRV has some limitations: It has a diminished capacity in identifying cavernous sinus and superficial cerebral veins thrombosis, partial thrombosis of other dural sinuses and cerebral veins, or net distinction between hypoplasia and occluded sinus [8].

Different MR techniques may be suitable to distinguish between sinus hypoplasia and dural sinus thrombosis. T2*GRE or T2*SWI MRI sequences will distinguish a normal signal in a hypoplastic sinus and an abnormally low signal in the occurrence of a thrombus [93–95]. Supplementary, a chronically thrombosed hypoplastic dural sinus will have absence of flow on 2D-TOF MRV and enhancement on CE-MRI and MRV [8].

CE-MRV sequences should be differentiated from different anatomical 3D T1 sequences, such as SPGR, BRAVO, TFE, and FFE [2].

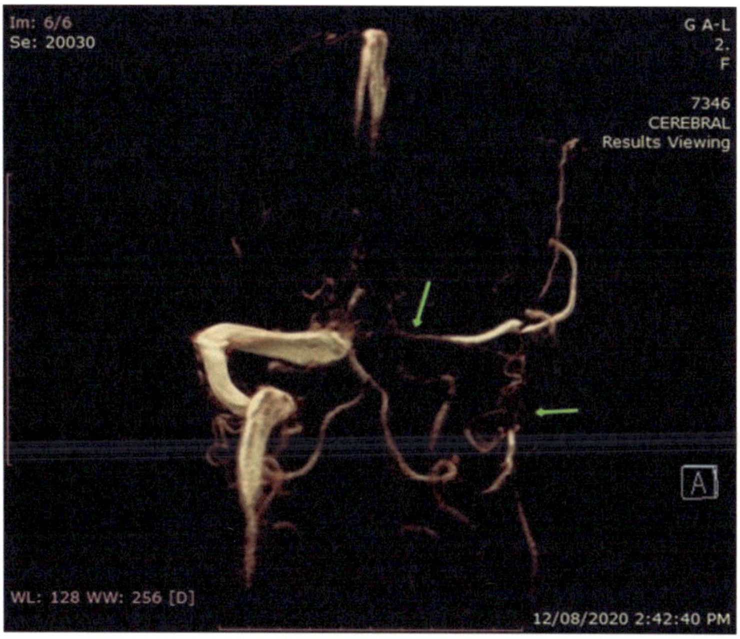

Figure 7.
3D-CORONAL VRT (reformatted by 2D-TOF venography) sequence shows an absent flow in left jugular bulb, left sigmoid sinus, left transverse sinus, and sinus confluence.

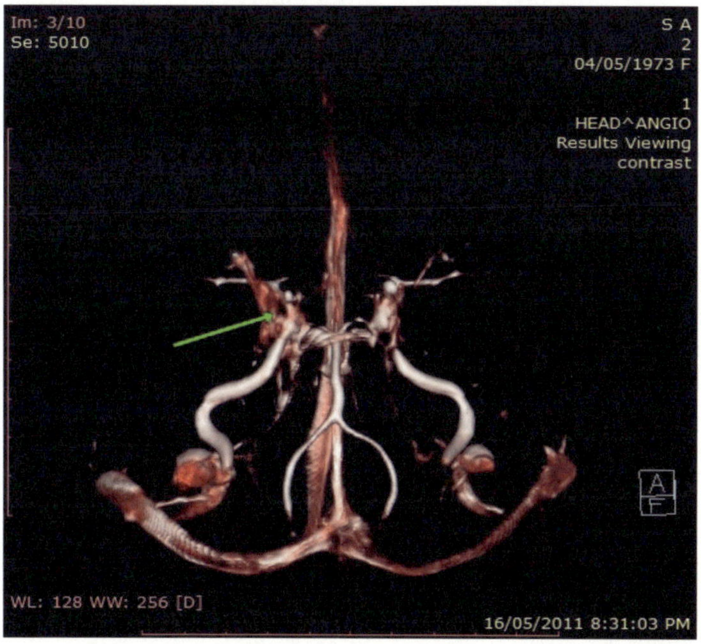

Figure 8.
3D-CORONAL VRT (reformatted by CE-MRA) sequence filling defect throughout the dural right cavernous sinus (arrow).

3D elliptical T1 post-gadolinium enhancement: It is a relatively newer technique, in which the paramagnetic effect of gadolinium shorts T1 and produces positive intravascular contrast enhancement [85, 98]. It realizes an improved assessment of the superficial and deep cerebral veins, and of the sinuses of the base of the skull (petrous, cavernous, and basilar plexus); an excellent detection of the lateral sinuses, even with hypoplasia; it overcomes the limitations of other MR techniques, especially signal losses in the situation of slow or turbulent flows (2D TOF, 2D, and 3D phase-contrast), not perpendicular to the acquisition plane (TOF) and in the event of unsuitable choice of encoding speed (2D and 3D phase-contrast) [85, 98].

3D phase-contrast (PC) MRV: It has a better capacity to detect slow flow and may better distinguish between slow flow and clot [97, 98]. Static contrast-enhanced 3D MRV detects better the cerebral veins and dural sinuses; unfortunately, it may present some restrictions in chronic dural sinus thrombosis as the clot may be enhanced, simulating a patent sinus [97, 98].

Time-resolved 3D MRV (4D MRV): This aspect is resolved with 4D MRV, which obtains images with diverse delays for better recognition of the venous clot [97]. This technique has better sensitivity to detect CVT than T2-WI, T2*GRE, and TOF-MRV; additionally, it has better specificity than TOF-MRV, and it recognizes better chronic CVT [97].

8.5 Cerebral intra-arterial angiography with venous phase imaging and direct cerebral venography

8.5.1 Cerebral intra-arterial angiography with venous phase imaging

It needs a four-vessel angiography (conventional or DSA) with detection of the whole venous phase on at least two projections (frontal and lateral) and three oblique views for the recognition on the entire SSS [14, 99].

Distinctive signs of CVT are represented by the following: partial deficiency of opacification or absence of filling of venous channels, late emptying, dilatation of cortical, scalp, or facial veins, dilatation of collateral veins, reverse of venous flow, and the abrupt ending of cortical veins encircled by tortuous and dilated collateral "corkscrew" veins [14, 99]. The obstruction of the posterior portion or the SSS, both LSs or the deep cerebral veins, is relatively easy to detect, but it can be misdiagnosed with hypoplasia or aplasia when the anterior third of the SSS or of the left LS is occluded [3, 14, 99]. Thus, we have to identify other imagistic features, such as occlusion of other cerebral vein or dural sinuses or delayed draining and dilatation of collateral veins in the occlusion of the anterior part of the SSS, or total absence of opacification of the whole sinus or its sigmoid segment in LS thrombosis, respectively [3]. This method presents some limitations: It does not detect the thrombus itself, and it is invasive, presents radiation exposure, possible allergy to the iodine contrast material, and requests teams of experts [3, 14, 99].

8.5.2 Direct cerebral venography

This technique is realized throughout endovascular therapeutic techniques, identifying the thrombus inside the venous channel either as an intra-vessel filling defect (no occlusive thrombosis) or as a complete no filling (occlusive thrombosis); complete obstruction by the clot may occur as a "cupping appearance" inside the dural sinus [14, 99]. Although the interobserver agreement for the detection of CVT is not excellent, the association of angiography with MRI will increase the interobserver agreement than angiography alone (94% versus 62%) [99].

9. Conclusions

CVT adult patients are younger, predominantly females, and have diminished frequencies of classical vascular risk factors when compared with cases with arterial infarcts.

The main risk factors for CVT in adults are prothrombotic conditions, either genetic or acquired.

The pathophysiology of CVT regulates the clinical picture and the abnormal imaging features. The nonspecific clinical spectrum of CVT may produce delays in diagnosis and consists of headache or intracranial hypertension, seizures, focal neurological deficits, and/or encephalopathy.

Both CT-CTV and MRI-MRV are outstanding methods to diagnose CVT and to distinguish consecutive complications. They may be associated with better evaluation.

Author details

Dragos Catalin Jianu[1,2,3]*, Silviana Nina Jianu[4], Nicoleta Iacob[5], Traian Flavius Dan[1,2,3], Georgiana Munteanu[1,2,3], Anca Elena Gogu[1,2,3] and Ligia Petrica[6]

1 First Division of Neurology, Department of Neurosciences-VIII, "Victor Babes" University of Medicine and Pharmacy, Timisoara, Romania

2 Centre for Cognitive Research in Neuropsychiatric Pathology (NeuroPsy-Cog), Department of Neurosciences, "Victor Babes" University of Medicine and Pharmacy, Timisoara, Romania

3 First Department of Neurology, "Pius Branzeu" Clinical Emergency County Hospital, Timisoara, Romania

4 Department of Ophthalmology, "Dr. Victor Popescu" Military Emergency Hospital, Timisoara, Romania

5 Department of Multidetector Computed Tomography and Magnetic Resonance Imaging, Neuromed Diagnostic Imaging Centre, Timisoara, Romania

6 Division of Nephrology, Department of Internal Medicine II, "Victor Babes", University of Medicine and Pharmacy, Timisoara, Romania

*Address all correspondence to: dcjianu@yahoo.com

References

[1] Jianu DC, Jianu SN, Dan TF, Munteanu G, Copil A, Birdac CD, et al. An integrated approach on the diagnosis of cerebral veins and Dural sinuses thrombosis (a narrative review). Life. 2022;**12**:717. DOI: 10.3390/life12050717

[2] Sadik JC, Jianu DC, Sadik R, Purcell Y, Novaes N, Saragoussi E, et al. Imaging of cerebral venous thrombosis. Life. 2022;**12**:1215. DOI: 10.3390/life12081215

[3] Mohr JP, Choi DW, Grotta JC, Weir B, Wolf PA. Stroke (Pathophysiology, Diagnosis, and Management). 4th ed. Philadelphia, Pennsylvania, USA: Churchill Livingstone; Chapter 12; 2004. pp. 301-325. DOI: 10.1016/B0-443-06600-0/X5001-9

[4] Stam J. Thrombosis of the cerebral veins and sinuses. The New England Journal of Medicine. 2005;**352**(17):1791-1798. PMID: 15858188. DOI: 10.1056/nejmra042354

[5] Piazza G. Cerebral venous thrombosis. Circulation. 2012;**125**:1704-1709. DOI: 10.1161/circulationaha.111.067835

[6] Dmytriw AA, Song JSA, Yu E, Poon CS. Cerebral venous thrombosis: State of the art diagnosis and management. Neuroradiology. 2018;**60**(7):669-685. DOI: 10.1007/s00234-018-2032-2

[7] Grotta JC, Albers GW, Broderick JP, Kasner SE, Lo EH, Mendelow AD, et al. Chapter 45: Cerebral venous thrombosis. In: Grotta JC, Albers GW, Broderick JP, Kasner SE, EH LO, Mendelow AD, Sacco RL, LKS W, editors. Stroke. 6th ed. Vol. 45. Newcastle, United Kingdom: Elsevier; 2016, 2016. pp. 716-730. DOI: 10.1016/B978-0-323-29544-4.00085-2

[8] Ferro JM, Canhão P. Cerebral venous thrombosis: Etiology, clinical features, and diagnosis. Newcastle, United Kingdom: UptoDate; 2023

[9] Ferro JM, Canhao P, Stam J, Bousser MG, Barinagarrementeria F. Prognosis of cerebral vein and dural sinus thrombosis: Results of the international study on cerebral vein and Dural sinus thrombosis (ISCVT). Stroke. 2004;**35**:664-670. DOI: 10.1161/01.str.0000117571.76197.26

[10] Caplan LR, Biller J, Leary MC, Lo EH, Thomas AJ, Yenari M, et al. Chapter 5: Anatomy of cerebral veins and Dural sinuses. In: Primer on Cerebrovascular Diseases. 2nd ed. Vol. 5. Cambridge, Massachusetts, USA: Academic Press; 2017. pp. 32-36. DOI: 10.1016/B978-0-12-803058-5.00005-9

[11] Satyarthee GD, Moscote-Salazar LR, Agrawal A. Persistent enlarged occipital sinus with absent unilateral transverse sinus. Journal of Neurosciences in Rural Practice. 2019;**10**:519-521. DOI: 10.1055/s-0039-1696081

[12] Valdueza JM, von Münster T, Hoffman O, Schreiber S, Einhäupl KM. Postural dependency of the cerebral venous outflow. The Lancet. 2000;**355**:200-201. DOI: 10.1016/s0140-6736(99)04804-7

[13] Coutinho JM, Zurbier SM, Aramideh M, Stam J. The incidence of cerebral venous thrombosis a cross-sectional study. Philadelphia, Pennsylvania, USA: Stroke. 2012;**43**:3375-3377. DOI: 10.1161/strokeaha.112.671453

[14] Saposnik G, Barinagarrementeria F, Brown RD Jr, Bushnell CD, Cucchiara B, Cushman M, et al. Diagnosis and management of cerebral venous thrombosis: A statement for healthcare professionals from

the American Heart Association/ American Stroke Association. Stroke. 2011;**42**(4):1158-1192. DOI: 10.1161/ str.0b013e31820a8364

[15] Coutinho JM, Ferro JM, Canhão P, Barinagarrementeria F, Cantú C, Bousser MG, et al. Cerebral venous and sinus thrombosis in women. Stroke. 2009 Jul;**40**(7):2356-2361. DOI: 10.1161/strokeaha.108.543884

[16] Devasagayam S, Wyatt B, Leyden J, Kleinig T. Cerebral venous sinus thrombosis incidence is higher than previously thought: A retrospective population-based study. Stroke. 2016;**47**:2180. DOI: 10.1161/ strokeaha.116.013617

[17] Ferro JM, Canhão P, Bousser MG, et al. Cerebral vein and dural sinus thrombosis in elderly patients. Stroke. 2005;**36**:1927. DOI: 10.1161/01. str.0000177894.05495.54

[18] Zuurbier SM, Hiltunen S, Lindgren E, et al. Cerebral venous thrombosis in older patients. Stroke. 2018;**49**:197. DOI: 10.1161/ strokeaha.117.019483

[19] deVeber G, Andrew M, Adams C, et al. Cerebral sinovenous thrombosis in children. The New England Journal of Medicine. 2001;**345**:417. DOI: 10.1056/ nejm200108093450604

[20] Marjot T, Yadav S, Hasan N, Bentley P, Sharma P. Genes associated with adult cerebral venous thrombosis. Stroke. 2011;**42**(4):913. DOI: 10.1161/ strokeaha.110.602672

[21] Lüdemann P, Nabavi DG, Junker R, Wolff E, Papke K, Buchner H, et al. Factor V Leiden mutation is a risk factor for cerebral venous thrombosis: A case-control study of 55 patients. Stroke. 1998;**29**(12):2507-2510. DOI: 10.1161/01. str.29.12.2507

[22] Weih M, Junge-Hülsing J, Mehraein S, Ziemer S, Einhäupl KM. Hereditary thrombophilia with ischemiC stroke and sinus thrombosis. Diagnosis, therapy and meta-analysis. Der Nervenarzt. 2000;**71**(12):936-945. DOI: 10.1007/s001150050690

[23] Biousse V, Conard J, Brouzes C, Horellou MH, Ameri A, Bousser MG. Frequency of the 20210 G –> a mutation in the 3′-untranslated region of the prothrombin gene in 35 cases of cerebral venous thrombosis. Stroke. 1998;**29**(7):1398-1400. DOI: 10.1161/01. str.29.7.1398

[24] Reuner KH, Ruf A, Grau A, Rickmann H, Stolz E, Jüttler E, et al. Prothrombin gene G20210 –> a transition is a risk factor for cerebral venous thrombosis. Stroke. 1998;**29**(9):1765-1769. DOI: 10.1161/01.str.29.9.1765

[25] Lauw MN, Barco S, Coutinho JM, Middeldorp S. Cerebral venous thrombosis and thrombophilia: A systematic review and meta-analysis. Seminars in Thrombosis and Hemostasis. 2013 Nov;**39**(8):913-927. DOI: 10.1055/s-0033-1357504

[26] Hillier CE, Collins PW, Bowen DJ, Bowley S, Wiles CM. Inherited prothrombotic risk factors and cerebral venous thrombosis. QJM. 1998;**91**(10):677-680. DOI: 10.1093/ qjmed/91.10.677

[27] Gouveia LO, Canhão P. MTHFR and the risk for cerebral venous thrombosis--a meta-analysis. Thrombosis Research. 2010;**125**(4):e153-e158. DOI: 10.1016/j.thromres.2009.10.019

[28] Gogu AE, Jianu DC, Dumitrascu V, Ples H, Stroe AZ, Docu Axelerad D, et al. MTHFR gene polymorphisms and cardiovascular risk Factors,Clinical-imagistic features and outcome in

cerebral venous sinus thrombosis. Brain Sciences. 2021;**11**(1):1-16. Article ID (number) 23. DOI: 10.3390/brainsci11010023

[29] Gogu AE, Motoc AG, Stroe AZ, Docu Axelerad A, Docu Axelerad D, Petrica L, et al. Plasminogen activator Inhibitor-1 (PAI-1) gene polymorphisms associated with cardio-vascular risk factors involved in cerebral venous sinus thrombosis. Metabolites. 2021;**11**(5):1-13. Article ID (number)266. DOI: 10.3390/metabo11050266

[30] Lee MK, Ng SC. Cerebral venous thrombosis associated with antithrombin III deficiency. Australian and New Zealand Journal of Medicine. 1991;**21**(5):772-773. DOI: 10.1111/j.1445-5994.1991.tb01388.x

[31] Deschiens MA, Conard J, Horellou MH, Ameri A, Preter M, Chedru F, et al. Coagulation studies, factor V Leiden, and anticardiolipin antibodies in 40 cases of cerebral venous thrombosis. Stroke. 1996;**27**(10):1724-1730. DOI: 10.1161/01.str.27.10.1724

[32] Duman T, Uluduz D, Midi I, Bektas H, Kablan Y, Goksel BK, et al. A Multicenter study of 1144 patients with cerebral venous thrombosis: The VENOST study. Journal of Stroke and Cerebrovascular Diseases. 2017;**26**(8):1848. DOI: 10.1016/j.jstrokecerebrovasdis.2017.04.020

[33] Ferro JM, Canhão P. Cerebral venous sinus thrombosis: Update on diagnosis and management. Current Cardiology Reports. 2014;**16**(9):523. DOI: 10.1007/s11886-014-0523-2

[34] Bousser MG, Crassard I. Cerebral venous thrombosis, pregnancy and oral contraceptives. Thrombosis Research. 2012;**130**(Suppl 1):S19-S22. DOI: 10.1016/j.thromres.2012.08.264

[35] Cantu C, Barinagarrementeria F. Cerebral venous thrombosis associated with pregnancy and puerperium. Review of 67 cases. Stroke. 1993;**24**(12):1880-1884. DOI: 10.1161/01.str.24.12.1880

[36] Lanska DJ, Kryscio RJ. Stroke and intracranial venous thrombosis during pregnancy and puerperium. Neurology. 1998;**51**(6):1622-1628. DOI: 10.1212/wnl.51.6.1622

[37] Kashkoush AI, Maa H, Agarwal N, Panczykowski D, Tonetti D, Weiner GM, et al. Cerebral venous sinus thrombosis in pregnancy and puerperium: A pooled, systematic review. Journal of Clinical Neuroscience. 2017;**39**:P9-P15. DOI: 10.1016/j.jocn.2017.02.046

[38] Martinelli I, Sacchi E, Landi G, Taioli E, Duca F, Mannucci PM. High risk of cerebral-vein thrombosis in carriers of a prothrombin-gene mutation and in users of oral contraceptives. The New England Journal of Medicine. 1998;**338**:1793-1797. DOI: 10.1056/nejm199806183382502

[39] de Bruijn SF, Stam J, Koopman MM, Vandenbroucke JP. Case-control study of risk of cerebral sinus thrombosis in oral contraceptive users and in [correction of who are carriers of hereditary prothrombotic conditions]. The cerebral venous sinus thrombosis study group. BMJ. 1998;**316**(7131):589-592. DOI: 10.1136/bmj.316.7131.589

[40] Zuurbier SM, Arnold M, Middeldorp S, et al. Risk of cerebral venous thrombosis in obese women. JAMA Neurology. 2016;**73**(5):579-584. DOI: 10.1001/jamaneurol.2016.0001

[41] Dentali F, Crowther M, Ageno W. Thrombophilic abnormalities, oral contraceptives, and risk of cerebral vein thrombosis: A meta-analysis. Blood. 2006;**107**(7):2766-2773. DOI: 10.1182/blood-2005-09-3578

[42] Knox AM, Brophy BP, Sage MR. Cerebral venous thrombosis in association with hormonal supplement therapy. Clinical Radiology. 1990;**41**(5):355-357. DOI: 10.1016/s0009-9260(05)81703-9

[43] Godeneche G, Gaillard N, Roy L, Mania A, Tondeur S, Chomel JC, et al. JAK2 V617F mutation associated with cerebral venous thrombosis: A report of five cases. Cerebrovascular Diseases. 2010;**29**(2):206-209. DOI: 10.1159/000267281

[44] Baldini T, Asioli GM, Romoli M, Carvalho Dias M, Schulte EC, Hauer L, et al. Cerebral venous thrombosis and severe acute respiratory syndrome coronavirus-2 infection: A systematic review and meta-analysis. European Journal of Neurology. 2021;**28**(10):3478-3490. DOI: 10.1111/ene.14727

[45] European Medicines Agency safety committee report. Available from: https://www.ema.europa.eu/en/news/astrazenecas-covid-19-vaccine-ema-finds-possible-link-very-rare-cases-unusual-blood-clots-low-blood [Accessed: 14, April 2021]

[46] Thakur KT, Tamborska A, Wood GK, McNeill E, David Roh D, Akpan IJ, et al. Clinical review of cerebral venous thrombosis in the context of COVID-19 vaccinations: Evaluation, management, and scientific questions. Journal of the Neurological Sciences. 2021;**427**:117532. DOI: 10.1016/j.jns.2021.117532

[47] Perry RJ, Tamborska A, Singh B, Craven B, Marigold R, Arthur-Farraj P, et al. Cerebral venous thrombosis after vaccination against COVID-19 in the UK: A multicenter cohort study. Lancet. 2021;**398**:1147-1156. DOI: 10.1016/s0140-6736(21)01608-1

[48] Pavord S, Scully M, Hunt BJ, Lester W, Bagot C, Craven B, et al. Clinical features of vaccine-induced immune thrombocytopenia and thrombosis. The New England Journal of Medicine. 2021;**385**(18):1680-1689. DOI: 10.1056/nejmoa2109908

[49] Greinacher A, Thiele T, Warkentin TE, Weisser K, Kyrle PA, EichingerS.Thromboticthrombocytopenia after ChAdOx1 nCov-19 vaccination. The New England Journal of Medicine. 2021;**384**(22):2092-2101. DOI: 10.1056/NEJMoa2104840

[50] Dobbs TD, Barber ZE, Squier WL, Green AL. Cerebral venous sinus thrombosis complicating traumatic head injury. Journal of Clinical Neuroscience. 2012;**19**(7):1058-1059. DOI: 10.1016/j.jocn.2012.01.002

[51] Schaller B, Graf R. Cerebral venous infarction-the pathophysiological concept. Cerebrovascular Diseases. 2004;**18**(3):179-188. DOI: 10.1159/000079939

[52] Gotoh M, Ohmoto T, Kuyama H. Experimental study of venous circulatory disturbance by dural sinus occlusion. Acta Neurochirurgica. 1993;**124**(2-4):120-126. DOI: 10.1007/bf01401133

[53] Lövblad KO, Bassetti C, Schneider J, Guzman R, El-Koussy M, Remonda L. Schroth G SO diffusion-weighted mr in cerebral venous thrombosis. Cerebrovascular Diseases. 2001;**11**(3):169-176. DOI: 10.1159/000047634

[54] Bousser MG, Chiras J, Bories J, Castaigne P. Cerebral venous thrombosis-a review of 38 cases. Stroke. 1985;**16**(2):199-213. DOI: 10.1161/01.str.16.2.199

[55] Ichord RN, Benedict SL, Chan AK, et al. Paediatric cerebral sinovenous thrombosis: Findings of the international

paediatric stroke study. Archives of Disease in Childhood. 2015;**100**:174. DOI: 10.1136/archdischild-2014-306382

[56] Biousse V, Ameri A, Bousser MG. Isolated intracranial hypertension as the only sign of cerebral venous thrombosis. Neurology. 1999;**53**(7):1537. DOI: 10.1212/wnl.53.7.1537

[57] Lopes MG, Ferro J, Pontes C, et al. Headache and cerebral venous thrombosis. Cephalalgia. 2000;**20**:292

[58] Cumurciuc R, Crassard I, Sarov M, et al. Headache as the only neurological sign of cerebral venous thrombosis: A series of 17 cases. Journal of Neurology, Neurosurgery, and Psychiatry. 2005;**76**:1084-1087. DOI: 10.1136/jnnp.2004.056275

[59] de Bruijn SF, Stam J, Kappelle LJ. Thunderclap headache as first symptom of cerebral venous sinus thrombosis. CVST study group. Lancet. 1996;**348**(9042):P1623-P1625. DOI: 10.1016/s0140-6736(96)07294-7

[60] Jianu DC, Jianu SN, Dan TF, Iacob N, Munteanu G, Motoc AGM, et al. Diagnosis and Management of Mixed Transcortical Aphasia due to multiple predisposing factors, including postpartum and severe inherited thrombophilia, affecting multiple cerebral venous and Dural sinus thrombosis: Case report and literature review. Diagnostics. 2021;**11**(8):1425. DOI: 10.3390/diagnostics11081425

[61] Ferro JM, Canhão P, Bousser MG, Stam J, Barinagarrementeria F. Early seizures in cerebral vein and Dural sinus thrombosis risk factors and role of Antiepileptics. Stroke. 2008;**39**:1152-1158. DOI: 10.1161/strokeaha.107.487363

[62] Ferro JM, Correia M, Rosas MJ, Pinto AN, Neves G, the Cerebral Venous Thrombosis Portuguese Collaborative Study Group [VENOPORT]. Seizures in cerebral vein and dural sinus thrombosis. Cerebrovascular Diseases. 2003;**15**:78-83. DOI: 10.1159/000067133

[63] Lancon JA, Killough KR, Tibbs RE, et al. Spontaneous dural sinus thrombosis in children. Pediatric Neurosurgery. 1999;**30**(1):23-29. DOI: 10.1159/000028755

[64] Ferro JM, Correia M, Pontes C, et al. Cerebral vein and dural sinus thrombosis in Portugal: 1980-1998. Cerebrovascular Diseases. 2001;**11**(3):177-182. DOI: 10.1159/000047635

[65] Damak M, Crassard I, Wolff V, Bousser MG. Isolated lateral sinus thrombosis a series of 62 patients. Stroke. 2009;**40**:476-481. DOI: 10.1161/strokeaha.107.509711

[66] Jianu DC, Jianu SN, Motoc AGM, Poenaru M, Petrica L, Vlad A, et al. Diagnosis and management of a young woman with acute isolated lateral sinus thrombosis. Romanian Journal of Morphology and Embryology. 2017;**58**(4):1515-1518 www.rjme.ro

[67] Waldvogel D, Mattle HP, Sturzenegger M, Schroth G. Pulsatile tinnitus--a review of 84 patients. Journal of Neurology. 1998;**245**(3):137-142. DOI: 10.1007/s004150050193

[68] Sakaida H, Kobayashi M, Ito A, Takeuchi K. Cavernous sinus thrombosis: Linking a swollen red eye and headache. Lancet. 2014;**384**(9946):928. DOI: 10.1016/s0140-6736(14)61404-5

[69] Ebright JR, Pace MT, Niazi AF. Septic thrombosis of the cavernous sinuses. Archives of Internal Medicine. 2001;**161**(22):2671-2676. DOI: 10.1001/archinte.161.22.2671

[70] Jacobs K, Moulin T, Bogousslavsky J, et al. The stroke syndrome of cortical vein thrombosis. Neurology. 1996;**47**(2):376-382. DOI: 10.1212/wnl.47.2.376

[71] Lacour JC, Ducrocq X, Anxionnat R, et al. Thrombosis of deep cerebral veins in form adults: Clinical features and diagnostic approach. Revue Neurologique (Paris). 2000;**156**(10):851-857

[72] van den Bergh WM, van der Schaaf I, van Gijn J. The spectrum of presentations of venous infarction caused by deep cerebral vein thrombosis. Neurology. 2005;**65**(2):192-196. DOI: 10.1212/01.wnl.0000179677.84785.63

[73] Pekçevik Y, Pekçevik R. Why should we report posterior fossa emissary veins? Diagnostic and Interventional Radiology. 2014;**20**(1):78-81. DOI: 10.5152/dir.2013.13203

[74] Jianu DC, Jianu SN, Dan TF, Motoc AGM, Poenaru M. Pulsatile tinnitus caused by a dilated left petrosquamosal sinus. Romanian Journal of Morphology and Embryology. 2016;**57**(1):319-322 www.rjme.ro

[75] Kuehnen J, Schwartz A, Neff W, Hennerici M. Cranial nerve syndrome in thrombosis of the transverse/sigmoid sinuses. Brain. 1998;**121**(Pt 2):381-388. DOI: 10.1093/brain/121.2.381

[76] Ferro JM, Bousser M-G, Canhãoa P, Coutinho JM, Crassard I, Dentali F, et al. European stroke organization guideline for the diagnosis and treatment of cerebral venous thrombosis – Endorsed by the European academy of neurology. European Journal of Neurology. 2017;**24**(10):1203-1213. DOI: 10.1111/ene.13381

[77] Dentali F, Squizzato A, Marchesi C, et al. D-dimer testing in the diagnosis of cerebral vein thrombosis: A systematic review and a meta-analysis of the literature. Journal of Thrombosis and Haemostasis. 2012;**10**(4):582-589. DOI: 10.1111/j.1538-7836.2012.04637.x

[78] Meng R, Wang X, Hussain M, et al. Evaluation of plasma D-dimer plus fibrinogen in predicting acute CVST. International Journal of Stroke. 2014;**9**(2):166-173. DOI: 10.1111/ijs.12034

[79] Canhão P, Abreu LF, Ferro JM, et al. Safety of lumbar puncture in patients with cerebral venous thrombosis. European Journal of Neurology. 2013;**20**(7):1075-1080. DOI: 10.1111/ene.12136

[80] Rizzo L, Crasto SG, Rudà R, et al. Cerebral venous thrombosis: Role of CT, MRI and MRA in the emergency setting. La Radiologia Medica. 2010;**115**(2):313-325. DOI: 10.1007/s11547-010-0493-4

[81] Qu H, Yang M. Early imaging characteristics of 62 cases of cerebral venous sinus thrombosis. Experimental and Therapeutic Medicine. 2013;**5**(1):233-236. DOI: 10.3892/etm.2012.796

[82] Boukobza M, Crassard I, Bousser MG, Chabriat H. MR imaging features of isolated cortical vein thrombosis: Diagnosis and follow-up. American Journal of Neuroradiology. 2009;**30**(2):344-348. DOI: 10.3174/ajnr.a1332

[83] Dan TF, Jianu SN, Iacob N, Motoc AGM, Munteanu G, Baloi A, et al. Management of an old woman with cavernous sinus thrombosis with two different mechanisms: Case report and review of the literature. Romanian Journal of Morphology and Embryology. 2020;**61**(4):1329-1334. DOI: 10.47162/RJME.61.4.35

[84] Buyck P-J, De Keyzer F, Vanneste D, Wilms G, Thijs V, Demaerel P. CT density

measurement and H:H ratio are useful in diagnosing acute cerebral venous sinus thrombosis. American Journal of Neuroradiology. 2013;**34**(8):1568-1572. DOI: 10.3174/ajnr.a3469

[85] Poon CS, Chang J-K, Swarnkar A, Johnson MH, Wasenko J. Radiologic diagnosis of cerebral venous thrombosis: Pictorial review. American Journal of Roentgenology. 2007;**189**(Suppl 6):S64-S75. DOI: 10.2214/ajr.07.7015

[86] Virapongse C, Cazenave C, Quisling R, et al. The empty delta sign: Frequency and significance in 76 cases of dural sinus thrombosis. Radiology. 1987;**162**(3):779-785. DOI: 10.1148/radiology.162.3.3809494

[87] Majoie CB, van Straten M, Venema HW, den Heeten GJ. Multisection CT venography of the dural sinuses and cerebral veins by using matched mask bone elimination. AJNR. American Journal of Neuroradiology. 2004;**25**:787 PMID: 15140721

[88] Khandelwal N, Agarwal A, Kochhar R, et al. Comparison of CT venography with MR venography in cerebral sinovenous thrombosis. AJR. American Journal of Roentgenology. 2006;**187**:1637. DOI: 10.2214/ajr.05.1249

[89] Leach JL, Fortuna RB, Jones BV, Gaskill-Shipley MF. Imaging of cerebral venous thrombosis: Current techniques, spectrum of findings, and diagnostic pitfalls. Radiographics. 2006;**26**(Suppl. 1): S19. DOI: 10.1148/rg.26si055174

[90] Rodallec MH, Krainik A, Feydy A, et al. Cerebral venous thrombosis and multidetector CT angiography: Tips and tricks. Radiographics. 2006;**26**(Suppl. 1): S5. DOI: 10.1148/rg.26si065505

[91] Dormont D, Anxionnat R, Evrard S, et al. MRI in cerebral venous thrombosis. Journal of Neuroradiology. 1994;**21**:81 PMID: 8014661

[92] Isensee C, Reul J, Thron A. Magnetic resonance imaging of thrombosed dural sinuses. Stroke. 1994;**25**:29. DOI: 10.1161/01.str.25.1.29

[93] Fellner FA, Fellner C, Aichner FT, Mölzer G. Importance of T2*-weighted gradient-echo MRI for diagnosis of cortical vein thrombosis. European Journal of Radiology. 2005;**56**:235. DOI: 10.1016/j.ejrad.2005.05.010

[94] Selim M, Fink J, Linfante I, et al. Diagnosis of cerebral venous thrombosis with echo-planar T2*-weighted magnetic resonance imaging. Archives of Neurology. 2002;**59**:1021. DOI: 10.1001/archneur.59.6.1021

[95] Mittal S, Wu Z, Neelavalli J, Haacke EM. Susceptibility weighted imaging: Technical aspects and clinical applications. Part 2. AJNR. American Journal of Neuroradiology. 2009;**30**:232-252. DOI: 10.3174/ajnr.A1461

[96] Favrole P, Guichard JP, Crassard I, et al. Diffusion-weighted imaging of intravascular clots in cerebral venous thrombosis. Stroke. 2004;**35**:99. DOI: 10.1161/01.str.0000106483.41458.af

[97] Meckel S, Reisinger C, Bremerich J, Damm D, Wolbers M, Engelter S, et al. Cerebral venous thrombosis: Diagnostic accuracy of combined, dynamic and static, contrast-enhanced 4D MR venography. AJNR. American Journal of Neuroradiology. 2010;**31**:527-535. DOI: 10.3174/ajnr.A1869

[98] Pallewatte AS, Tharmalingam T, Liyanage N. Anatomic variants and artefacts in non-enhanced MRV - potential pitfalls in diagnosing cerebral venous sinus thrombosis (CVST). SLJR.

2016;**2**(1):40-46. DOI: 10.4038/sljr.v2i1.23

[99] Wetzel SG, Kirsch E, Stock KW, et al. Cerebral veins: Comparative study of CT venography with intraarterial digital subtraction angiography. AJNR. American Journal of Neuroradiology. 1999;**20**:249 PMCID: PMC7056122

Chapter 6

Action on the Cerebral Vascular Endothelium in the Prevention of Stroke

Andrés J. Ursa Herguedas and María Pellón Olmedo

Abstract

Stroke or cerebrovascular accident (CVA) is a frequent, disabling pathology, consumes enormous social and health resources and has high morbidity and mortality. A large part of the resources of the health systems are allocated to the treatment of stroke, which is achieving better results every time, and far fewer resources are allocated to prevention. The objective of this review is to raise awareness in the different states so that they allocate more resources to prevention through awareness programs for health personnel, and implementation of detection tests for atherosclerotic cardiovascular disease in order to reduce the incidence of stroke. Clients should be insisted on adopting an adequate lifestyle, as well as acting on risk factors. Most strokes can be prevented through health education, blood pressure control, and lifestyle changes such as eating a healthy diet, being physically active, and stopping smoking.

Keywords: prevention of stroke or cerebrovascular accident, atherosclerotic cardiovascular disease, endothelial dysfunction, cerebrovascular diseases, gut dysbiosis

1. Introduction

Atherosclerotic cardiovascular disease (ACVD) is a chronic, generalized, and progressive pathology that modifies the arteries until it causes a cardiovascular event. Elevated low-density lipoproteins (LDL-C) in plasma over time is one of the main causes of this disease, along with other risk factors. Cardiovascular diseases are the leading cause of disability and death from middle ages of life in developed countries, in both sexes. Cerebrovascular disease (CVD) encompasses anatomoclinical entities caused by reduced blood supply in a certain vascular territory (ischemic-type CVD) or by rupture of an intracranial vessel (hemorrhagic-type CVD) [1].

One in six people in the world will suffer a stroke, representing the third cause of death in the West, being the first in women. In Europe, 1.3 million people suffer a stroke each year and it is the second most frequent cause of death. With about 25 million cases per year, acute ischemic stroke represents a major public health challenge worldwide [2, 3]. Strokes have increased globally in absolute terms, as well as associated deaths, partly due to the greater number of cases registered in low- and middle-income countries as well as the aging of the population [4]. In total, 90% of stroke cases can be correlated with behavioral factors, including poor diet, smoking, and little physical activity, as well as metabolic factors such as obesity, hypertension, and diabetes mellitus [5].

The four main noncommunicable diseases (NCDs), such as cardiovascular disease (including stroke), cancer, type 2 diabetes mellitus (DM2), and lung disease, share 4 risk factors: tobacco use, unhealthy diet, physical inactivity, and alcohol abuse. Therefore, from a public health perspective, mass actions on lifestyle factors are the most cost-effective means of NCD prevention [6]. In recent years, several studies have reported that alterations in the gut microbiota (GM) could be a risk factor for stroke [7, 8]. Vascular endothelial dysfunction (VED) presents with a loss of balance between the vasodilation and vasoconstriction factors derived from it, with a predominance of the latter, producing progressive pathophysiological changes that make it possible to cause proinflammatory, prooxidant, proliferative, and procoagulant effects and vascular adhesion, contributing to atherogenesis in each of its phases [9].

The prevention of ACVD in high-risk patients is one of the main challenges that healthcare professionals face in order to reduce the rates of morbidity and mortality from stroke.

Primary prevention refers to the adoption of a healthy lifestyle from an early age and secondary prevention refers to the implementation of measures aimed at acting on cardiovascular risk factors (CVRF).

2. Causal factors

Ischemic infarcts are produced by the acute occlusion of one of the large cervical or cerebral arteries, either by a gradual narrowing of atherosclerotic origin or by a sudden occlusion produced by a thrombus (if it originates from the same cerebral arterial system) or an embolus (if the clot originates in a region of the vascular system other than the brain). In the case of hemorrhagic stroke, the rupture of a blood vessel occurs either at the intracerebral level (intracerebral hemorrhage) or by the rupture of aneurysms at the bifurcation of the great arteries on the surface of the brain (subarachnoid hemorrhage). Most strokes are ischemic (85%) and 15% hemorrhagic. A total of 15% of strokes occur in children [10, 11]. A small percentage of ACVD is related to genes [12].

Different studies demonstrated an association between elevated levels of total cholesterol and LDL-C and increased risk of ischemic stroke [13, 14]. A high intake of sugars, including added sugars and those naturally present in honey and fruit juices, is associated with an increased risk of developing cardiovascular diseases and, specifically, stroke [15]. In recent years, several studies have linked stroke with gut dysbiosis (GD) [16]. Although there are many causes of stroke, this chapter focuses on the prevention of ischemic strokes as they are the most frequent.

3. Ischemic stroke risk factors

Most strokes are due to modifiable risk factors, so there is a possibility of prevention. The main non-modifiable risk factor for stroke is age. In one-third of strokes, the cause is unknown [17].

Table 1 contains the most frequent modifiable risk factors according to O'Donnell et al., [18], updated by the authors.

Potentials	Established
Obesity/overweight	High blood pressure
Sedentary lifestyle	Diabetes mellitus
Glucose intolerance	Carotid stenosis
Malnutrition	Atrial fibrillation
Excessive alcohol intake	Previous ischemic heart disease
Smoking	Smoking
Blood hypercoagulable states	Sickle cell anemia
Hyperhomocysteinemia	
Drug addiction (cocaine, etc.)	
Use of oral contraceptives/Hormone replacement therapy	
Inflammatory processes	
Obstructive sleep apnea	
Intestinal dysbiosis, alteration of the intestinal barrier, and neuroinflammation	

Table 1.
Modifiable risk factors in stroke prevention according to O'Donnell et al., 2016 [18], updated by the authors.

Arterial hypertension (AHT) is the main risk factor involved in cerebrovascular disease, both in ischemic and hemorrhagic strokes. GD has been observed in the prehypertensive state compared to a normotensive population. These changes precede the development of AHT and are not due to AHT itself [19]. Obesity increases the risk of suffering a stroke, especially abdominal fat. It is a public health problem because it is related to many diseases, among others, hypertension and DM2. Furthermore, the number of cases has increased greatly in recent years and has become an epidemic [20]. A sedentary lifestyle, as a cardiometabolic risk factor, contributes to the appearance of a stroke [21]. The cardiovascular risk in patients with obesity and DM2 is increased since it is generally accompanied by other cardiovascular risk factors such as AHT, hypercholesterolemia, hypertriglyceridemia, and metabolic syndrome (MS) among others [22, 23]. For several decades, numerous studies have linked the act of smoking with an increased risk of stroke. The related components are attributed to nicotine, oxidizing gases, and carbon monoxide. This risk also exists in passive smokers [24]. According to the 2016 Interstroke study, high and moderate alcohol intake is associated with an increased chance of suffering a stroke [18]. Prediabetes and DM2 are associated with increased vascular risk in parallel with the degree of hyperglycemia and the lack of good metabolic control. In patients with type 1 diabetes mellitus, the frequency of stroke is lower. Diabetics are at high risk of atherosclerosis and often have other atherogenic risk factors, such as AHT, hyperlipidemia, and obesity, known as MS [25]. The role of dyslipidemias, especially the elevation of total serum cholesterol, as well as LDL-C is a known factor in CVD that contributes to ischemic stroke [13, 14]. Established AHT is one of the most prevalent modifiable risk factors, being associated with more severe strokes and with a worse prognosis [26]. The causal relationship between GM and AHT is more evident when studying AHT secondary to obstructive sleep apnea syndrome [27]. The presence of a coagulopathy is a potential risk factor for a cardiovascular event, but another independent risk factor is necessary, which acts by another mechanism to predispose to strokes, such as taking oral contraceptives, homocystinuria, etc. [28].

Associated with the aging process, there is a loss in the integrity of the intestinal epithelial barrier, a decrease in the number of enteric neurons and an increase in the synthesis of proinflammatory cytokines [29], factors possibly involved in the higher incidence of stroke from the average age of life.

4. Role of the microbiota-gut-brain axis in cerebrovascular disease

In the intestine, a series of products are generated by GM that exert their influence on the central nervous system (CNS), such as short-chain fatty acids (SCFAs), secondary bile acids, or tryptophan metabolites, which exert their function through ascending signals that start locally, either by crossing the intestinal barrier to pass into the systemic circulation or even acting directly in the CNS by crossing the blood-brain barrier [30]. Microbial products that reach systemic circulation are capable of modulating the immune system toward a more inflammatory environment or inducing tolerance, both locally and in the CNS. A central role in this modulation is exerted through the products generated by the metabolism of dietary components, such as dietary fiber, tryptophan, or arginine, which give rise to polyamines, indoles, and SCFA, which are capable of increasing the expansion of regulatory T lymphocytes, favoring an antiinflammatory phenotype in dendritic cells and decreasing the production of proinflammatory cytokines in neutrophils and macrophages. Another mechanism that GM also uses to regulate the immune response is the modification of the host's own metabolites, in the case of secondary bile acids that regulate dendritic cells, macrophages, and natural killer cells, or through metabolites produced by intestinal bacteria, such as polysaccharide A from Bacteroides fragilis, with an antiinflammatory effect, or those produced by segmented filamentous bacteria, with a proinflammatory effect [31]. On the other hand, a correlation has been found between the increased risk of stroke and a greater burden of opportunistic pathogens, together with low levels of butyrate-producing intestinal bacteria [32]. Recent studies in animal models and later in human fecal samples after suffering an ischemic stroke compared to a control group have linked a certain GM with a higher risk of suffering a stroke, so it would become a modifiable risk factor [33]. Currently, the actions of microorganisms are beginning to be assessed as risk factors, such as infections caused by Chlamydia pneumoniae and Helicobacter pylori, reactivation of the varicella-zoster virus, etc. [34].

Within the actions of the microbiota-gut-brain axis (MGBA), through the vagus nerve, different microbial metabolites are detected and are capable of generating responses at the central level, as well as producing cholinergic responses secondary to peripheral inflammation, which translate into alterations in intestinal permeability and modulation of GM composition [35]. Among the environmental factors that increase intestinal permeability are alcohol consumption, prolonged use of antibiotics, abuse of non-steroidal antiinflammatory drugs, food allergies, radiation, and chemotherapy. Another group is made up of artificial sweeteners, such as aspartame and sucralose, pesticides, some household detergents, environmental pollutants, gluten in celiac patients, and the consumption of some marine fish that concentrate heavy metals [36, 37]. Under certain circumstances, GM can become unbalanced and favor the expansion of pathobiont microorganisms, organisms of the GM that are harmless under normal conditions but with infectious capacity in certain states [38], which can alter the entire host immune response and increase permeability of bowel [37]. Large uncharged molecules, such as proteins or lipopolysaccharides, or large charged molecules can pass through the tight junctions between epithelial cells [39]. However, deregulation of these junctions as a result of genetic or environmental factors, such as diet, drug use, or the activity of pathogenic microorganisms, can cause increased intestinal permeability. This phenomenon is frequently observed in inflammatory bowel diseases and in some metabolic diseases, such as diabetes or obesity [40]. In murine models, it has been observed that GM is a factor that can significantly influence the genesis of stroke [41]. SCFAs are an important class of bacterial metabolites that are obtained from the fermentation of polysaccharides (fibers) [42]. Preliminary studies showed that SCFAs have an important role in maintaining intestinal integrity and have an antiinflammatory effect [43]. One of the SCFAs, butyrate, is a preferential energy source for intestinal epithelial cells, thus contributing to their physiology [44]. SCFAs can reach the brain, due to the presence of transporters of these molecules in the endothelial cells of the blood-brain barrier [45]. Once there, they can modulate neuroinflammation by acting on the morphology and activation of microglia in the event of stroke [45].

GM can generate potentially toxic compounds, such as the formation of trimethylamine from choline and carnitine present in the diet [46]. Trimethylamine is absorbed and transformed into trimethylamine N-oxide (TMAO) in the liver, being considered a risk factor for cardiovascular disease [47].

These mechanisms may partly explain the factors dependent on the human microbiome that may favor stroke.

5. Role of the vascular endothelium

Endothelial cells (ECs) are capable of detecting physical changes related to mechanical stress caused by blood flow, blood pressure, or wall distension. When an imbalance occurs in the bioavailability of vasoactive substances, the predisposition to platelet aggregation, thrombosis, inflammation, vasoconstriction, or increased vascular permeability, a situation called vascular endothelial dysfunction (VED), occur.

VED is one of the initial events of atherosclerosis, it plays a fundamental role in ACVD and, therefore, in CVD [48]. GM has the ability to produce metabolites that directly affect the host's cardiovascular system, being able to generate antagonistic effects (pro- and antiinflammatory, vasodilator, and vasoconstrictor) with both beneficial and harmful results. These metabolites include SCFA, TMAO, nitrites, indoles, and hydrogen sulfide. In AHT models, it has been shown that there is a decrease in the intestinal bacterial populations that produce SCFA and hydrogen sulfide (both with vasodilator properties). At the other extreme, TMAO-type metabolites, as well as indoles, would favor arterial vasoconstriction [49]. In experimental animals, it has been possible to induce atherosclerotic lesions similar to those found in human arteries, through the administration of diets rich in cholesterol and saturated fat. This type of diet produces an increase in plasma LDL-C concentrations and facilitates its accumulation in the subendothelial space in areas where permeability is increased. In these models, it has been observed that the regions most prone to developing atherosclerotic lesions present a greater permeability to LDL-C and very low-density lipoproteins (VLDL) [50]. It has been observed that high concentrations of native LDL-C and low concentrations of oxidized LDL-C increase vascular permeability since they reduce the content of heparan sulfate proteoglycans in the extracellular matrix of the subendothelial space. This effect would be produced by a negative regulation of the synthesis of these molecules, as well as an increase in their degradation thanks to the induction of endothelial secretion of heparanase [51].

VED is characterized by an imbalance between the relaxation and contraction factors derived from the endothelium [52] and is both the cause and effect of atherosclerotic lesions in cerebral arteries [53]. In SARS-Cov-2 infection, thrombotic complications are frequent and severe. Loss of even a small number of endothelial cells due to infection could lead to a breakdown of the endothelial barrier, resulting in "vascular leakage," thus exposing inflammatory cells. This would lead to an abnormal activation of the coagulation system that would cause inflammation of small vessels and microthrombi, which could affect the heart, lungs, or brain [54].

Numerous factors and markers of endothelial damage have been studied, which turn out to be predictors of an advance in the development of atherosclerotic plaque and, therefore, of its instability. The quantification of the degree of vasodilation mediated by hyperflow (VMH) of the brachial artery is a noninvasive, cheap, simple, reproducible, readily available, and validated ultrasonographic technique that allows us to know the state of health and function of the vascular endothelium. It is a response dependent on endothelial nitric oxide and, when it is decreased, translates to a VED. VMH is reduced in patients with vascular risk factors, cerebral, coronary, or peripheral vascular disease, and is an independent predictor of vascular events and vascular recurrence. It also allows us to be able to detect and quantify the degree of VED early, anticipating the appearance of atheromatous plaque. VED improves with various drugs, such as antihypertensives, antidiabetics, antiaggregants, or lipid-lowering agents [55].

6. Precautionary measures

Stroke is a disease that, to a large extent, can be avoided. Therefore, identifying the risk factors of each person is key to drawing up a preventive strategy at the individual level. The scope of action to carry out these activities is primary health care. A healthy lifestyle can reduce the risk of cardiovascular events. Most strokes can be prevented with hygienic-dietary habits. For this, modifiable risk factors must be monitored, such as obesity/overweight, sedentary lifestyle, smoking, alcohol abuse, AHT, dyslipidemia, DM2, and previous heart disease. There are cardiovascular risk factors that cannot be modified, such as age, sex, family history, thrombophilia, and previous strokes. It is necessary to carry out awareness campaigns on stroke in preventive aspects. **Table 2** contains the recommendations of the Diabetes and Cardiovascular Disease Working Group of the Spanish Diabetes Society (SED, 2014–2015) [22].

Eating a healthy diet, rich in plant-based foods, can help modify IM so that the production of deleterious metabolites such as TMAO is reduced [56]. Plant-based diets are associated with significant benefits in the improvement or prevention of metabolic diseases (overweight, obesity, DM2), cardiovascular disease, inflammatory bowel disease, and chronic kidney disease. In addition, a very important emerging aspect, in which the evidence is growing, is the beneficial effect on aging and aspects linked to it, such as sarcopenia [57, 58]. Proteins, carbohydrates, and fats present in plant foods can shift the GM profile toward increased production of antiinflammatory compounds and decreased production of endogenous toxins. Vegetable fats, particularly olive oil, are antiinflammatory and antiatherogenic [21].

Aspects to consider	Recommendations	Intervention
Mediterranean diet	Diet with a predominance of plant-based foods	Celiacs, food allergies, and intolerances
Physical exercise	Aerobic, 150 minutes a week, 3 days minimum with moderate intensity.	Adaptations according to particular situation
Quitting the smoking habit	Collect in the medical history the beginning, frequency of consumption, if you inhale smoke, etc.	Choosing the most appropriate smoking cessation method
Overweight/obesity	Progressive weight loss until reaching ideal weight	BMI >35 + DM2: bariatric surgery
Glycemic control	Hb1c < 7	Hb1c >8 + CVFR, DM2, elderly, complications, etc.
Lipids	LDL-C < 100 mg/dl (Primary prevention) LDL-C < 70 mg/dl (secondary prevention)	Diet + physical exercise Statins etc.
Blood pressure	< 140/90 mmHg low salt diet	In case of nephropathy: Angiotensin-converting enzyme inhibitors, etc.
Blood coagulation status	Primary and secondary prevention	Acetylsalicylic acid: 100 mg/day in case of CVFR
Vitamins	Vitamin D > 30 ng/ml Vitamin B12 > 160 pg./ml	Supplement with levels <20 ng/ml Supplement in case of prescription of metformin, vegan diet

Table 2.
Recommendations of the diabetes and cardiovascular disease working group (SED, 2014–2015), adapted by the authors of the chapter.

Moderate-intensity physical exercise, such as walking or cycling, should be part of daily activity in healthy adults [59, 60]. Keeping your weight within healthy limits is very important for the normal functioning of the heart, blood vessels, metabolism, bones, and other organs. All this happens to maintain a balance between the calories that are ingested. A balanced diet, physical exercise, and in some cases drugs can help achieve this goal. Glycemic control, especially in predisposed patients, is an important factor in order to prevent the complications of DM2. Various antidiabetic drugs may play an important role in stroke prevention [61]. The management of dyslipidemias is based on implementing healthy lifestyle habits and pharmacological treatment. The indication to start lipid-lowering treatment will depend on the vascular risk of each subject. Statins are the drugs of choice. Other effective lipid-lowering agents are ezetimibe combined with statins and PCSK9 (protein convertase subtilisin-kexin type 9) inhibitors. Other drugs such as fibrates or omega-3 fatty acids are useful in the management of triglycerides, although their usefulness in the prevention of vascular diseases is not well defined [62, 63]. Reducing blood pressure is the key, both in the primary prevention of the disease and in the secondary to avoid its recurrence. It is recommended to start antihypertensive treatment for primary prevention of stroke in patients with blood pressure figures higher than 140/90 mmHg [26]. Anticoagulants are recommended in case of atrial fibrillation in any patient over 75 years of age and with several CVRFs [64].

In stroke prevention campaigns, emphasis must be placed on the importance of rapid action in the event of a stroke. Hospitals have protocols (stroke code) for early diagnosis with imaging tests using artificial intelligence and early treatment in order to minimize neurological damage. Having suffered a stroke is a risk factor for suffering it again. For this reason, secondary prevention, the adoption of good lifestyle habits, and good adherence to prescribed treatments are essential [65]. Once the sequelae of the stroke have been assessed early, both physical (speech therapy and physiotherapy) as well as social and psychological rehabilitation begins after 48–72 hours. The idea is to go to a neurorehabilitation unit. The objective is for the patient to remain independent and autonomous for the basic and instrumented activities of daily life. Between 40 and 50% of patients abandon treatment 2 or 3 years after having suffered a stroke, which favors the appearance of a second event, the repercussion of which will be worse than that of the first [66]. Biomarkers that predict stroke outcome include serum triglyceride level, HDL-cholesterol [67], interleukin-6 (IL-6), NT-proBNP [68], and YKL-40 [69]. IM modulation, especially with prebiotics and/or probiotics, represents a preventive and therapeutic approach to take into account in the approach to ACVD [70].

7. Conclusions

1. The adoption of a lifestyle based on a diet with a predominance of foods of vegetable origin and the performance of physical exercise adapted according to age is the basis for the prevention of atherosclerotic cardiovascular disease.

2. In primary prevention, it is recommended to determine the patient's vascular risk in order to define the appropriate LDL-C figure.

3. In secondary prevention after a stroke of atherothrombotic origin, LDL-C levels of less than 55 mg/dl are recommended, while in ischemic strokes of nonatherothrombotic origin, the objectives will be established based on the vascular risk group of each patient.

4. Both in primary and secondary prevention, statins are the drugs of first choice in dyslipidemia, and ezetimibe and/or PCSK9 inhibitors can be associated in those cases that do not reach the therapeutic objectives.

5. In the near future, we will be able to prevent strokes or improve neurological recovery through intervention in the gut microbiota.

Acknowledgements

The chapter has been funded by the Institute for Integrative Medicine.

Conflict of interest

There is no conflict of interest.

Abbreviations

CVA	cerebrovascular accident or stroke
ACVD	atherosclerotic cardiovascular disease
CVD	cerebrovascular disease
NCD	noncommunicable diseases
DM 2	type 2 diabetes mellitus
GM	gut microbiota
VED	vascular endothelial dysfunction
CVRF	cardiovascular risk factors
LDL-C	low-density lipoproteins
GD	gut dysbiosis
AHT	arterial hypertension
MS	metabolic syndrome
CNS	central nervous system
SCFAs	short chain fatty acids
MGBA	microbiota-gut-brain axis
EC	endothelial cells
TMAO	trimethylamine oxide
VLDL	very low-density lipoproteins
VMH	quantification of the degree of vasodilatation mediated by hyperflow
IL-6	interleukin 6

Author details

Andrés J. Ursa Herguedas[1,2,3,4,5,6,7]* and María Pellón Olmedo[8,9,10,11,12,13,14]

1 Institute of Integrative Medicine, Valladolid, Spain

2 Complutense University of Madrid, Madrid, Spain

3 Junta de Castilla y León, Valladolid, Spain

4 Rehabilitation and Pain from the University of Valladolid, Spain

5 Clinical Neurophysiology from the University of Valladolid, Spain

6 Academy of Health Sciences Dr. Ramón y Cajal, Madrid, Spain

7 Dr. Gómez Ulla Award for Health Excellence, Madrid, Spain

8 Pharmacy from the University of Salamanca, Spain

9 Human Nutrition and Dietetics from the University of Valladolid, Spain

10 Pharmacy from the University of Valladolid, Spain

11 University and Non-University Education (health area), Spain

12 Pharmaceutical Care from the University of Valencia, Spain

13 Orthopedics and Technical Aids from the University of Salamanca, Spain

14 CESME (Faculty of Medicine of Valladolid) and of the SEFAC Nutrition Group, Spain

*Address all correspondence to: ajursa@educa.jcyl.es

References

[1] Torregrosa G et al. Basic pathophysiology: From arterial occlusion to neuronal death. In: Montaner J, editor. Pathophysiology of Cerebral Ischemia. Barcelona, Spain: ICG Marge. SL; 2007. pp. 13-31

[2] Purroy F, Montalá N. Epidemiology of stroke in the last decade. Neurology Journal. 2021;**73**(9):321-336. DOI: 10.33588/rn.7309.2021138

[3] Feigin VL, Norrving B, Mensah GA. Global burden of stroke. Circulation Research. 2017;**120**(3):439-448. DOI: 10.1161/CIRCRESAHA.116.308413

[4] Katan M, Luft A. Global burden of stroke. Seminars in Neurology. 2018;**38**(02):208-211. DOI: 10.1055/s-0038-1649503

[5] Hernández Ruiz de Eguilaz M, Batlle MA, Martínez de Morentin B, San-Cristóbal R, Pérez-Díez S, Navas-Carretero S, et al. Dietary and lifestyle changes as a strategy in the prevention of metabolic syndrome and type 2 diabetes mellitus: Milestones and perspectives. Annals of the Navarrese Health System. 2016 (cited 2023 Mar 27);**39**(2):269-289 Available from: http://scielo.isciii.es/scielo.php?script=sci_arttext&pid=S1137-66272016000200009&lng=es

[6] Beaglehole R, Bonita R, Horton R, Adams C, Alleyne G, Asaria P, et al. Priority actions for the non-communicable disease crisis. Lancet. 2011;**377**(9775):1438-1447. DOI: 10.1016/S0140-6736(11)60393-0

[7] Li H, Zhang X, Pan D, Liu Y, Yan X, Tang Y, et al. Dysbiosis characteristics of gut microbiota in cerebral infarction patients. Translational Neuroscience. 2020;**11**(1):124-133. DOI: 10.1515/tnsci-2020-6117. Available from: https://www.degruyter.com/document/doi/10.1515/tnsci-2020-0117/html

[8] Rodríguez Perón JM, Rodríguez Izquierdo MM. Bioactive metabolites generated by intestinal dysbiosis and their pathophysiological implications in cardiovascular disease. Revista Cubana de Medicina. 2022;**61**(1):e2584 Available from: http://scielo.sld.cu/scielo.php?script=sci_arttext&pid=S0034-75232022000100013&lng=es

[9] Carvajal Carvajal C. The endothelium: Structure, function and endothelial dysfunction. Legal Medicine of Costa Rica. virtual edition. 2017;**34**(2):90-100 ISSN 2215-5287

[10] Diez-Tejedor E, del Brutto O, Alvarez Sabin J, et al. Classification of cerebrovascular diseases. Iberoamerican Society of Cerebrovascular Diseases Neurology Magazine. 2001;**33**:455-456. DOI: 10.33588/rn.3305.2001246

[11] Sobrino García P, García Pastor A, García Arratibel A, Vicente Peracho G, Rodríguez Cruz PM, Pérez Sánchez JR, et al. Etiological classification of ischemic stroke: Comparison between the new A-S-C-O classification and the classification of the study Group of Cerebrovascular Diseases of the Spanish Society of Neurology. Neurology. 2013;**28**(7):417-424. DOI: 10.1016/j.nrl.2012.07.005

[12] Chauhan G, Debette S. Genetic risk factors for ischemic and hemorrhagic stroke. Current Cardiology Reports. 2016;**18**(12):124. DOI: 10.1007/s11886-016-0804-z

[13] Yaghi S, Elkind MS. Lipids and cerebrovascular disease. Research and

Practice. Stroke. 2015;**46**:3322-3328. DOI: 10.1161/estrokeaha.115.011164

[14] Lee JS, Chang PY, Zhang Y, Kizer JR, Best LG, Howard BV. Triglyceride and HDL-C dyslipidemia and risks of coronary heart disease and ischemic stroke by glycemic dysregulation status: The strong heart study. Diabetes Care. 2017;**40**(4):529-537. DOI: 10.2337/dc16-1958

[15] Kelly RK et al. Associations between types and sources of dietary carbohydrates and cardiovascular disease risk: A prospective cohort study of UK biobank participants. BMC Medicine. 2023;**21**:34. DOI: 10.1186/s12916-022-02712-7

[16] Zeng X, Gao X, Peng Y, Wu Q, Zhu J, Tan C, et al. Higher risk of stroke is correlated with increased opportunistic pathogen load and reduced levels of butyrate-producing bacteria in the gut. Frontiers in Cellular and Infection Microbiology. 2019;**9**:4. DOI: 10.3389/fcimb.2019.00004

[17] O'Donnell MJ, Javier D, Liu L, et al. Risk factors for intracerebral and ischemic hemorrhagic stroke in 22 countries (the INTERSTROKE study): A case-control study. Lancet. 2010;**376**:112-123. DOI: 10.1016/S0140-6736(10)60834-3

[18] O'Donnell MJ et al. Global and regional effects of potentially modifiable risk factors associated with acute stroke in 32 countries (INTERSTROKE): A case-control study. Lancet. 2016;**388**:761-775. DOI: 10.1016/S0140-6736(16)30506-2

[19] Arredondo Bruce A, Guerrero Jiménez G, Arredondo RA. Relationship between intestinal microbiota and blood pressure. MEDISAN. 2019;**23**(5):967-980 Available from: http://scielo.sld.cu/scielo.php?script=sci_arttext&pid=S1029-30192019000500967&lng=es

[20] Rodríguez-Campello A, Jiménez-Conde J, Ois Á, Cuadrado-Godia E, Giralt-Steinhauer E, Vivanco RM, et al. Sex-related differences in abdominal obesity impact on ischemic stroke risk. European Journal of Neurology. 2016;**24**(2):1-7. DOI: 10.1111/ene.13216

[21] Arocha RJI. Cardiometabolic risk of sedentary lifestyle. Clinical Hospital University of Chile Magazine. 2023;**32**(3) Retrieved from: https://revistahospitalclinico.uchile.cl/index.php/RHCUC/article/view/69536

[22] Arrieta F et al. Diabetes mellitus and cardiovascular risk: Recommendations of the diabetes and cardiovascular disease working Group of the Spanish Diabetes Society (SED, 2015). Primary Care. 2016;**48**(5):325-336. DOI: 10.1016/j.aprim.2015.05.002

[23] Muñoz Roldán I, Martín Puig M, Agudo Villa M, Recarte García C, Millán J. Cardiovascular risk in type 2 diabetic patients with or without associated metabolic syndrome. Clinic and research in arteriosclerosis. 2011;**23**(3):112-118. DOI: 10.1016/j.arteri.2011.03.002

[24] Bonita R, Scragg R, Stewart A, Jackson R, Beaglehole R. Cigarette smoking and risk of premature stroke in men and women. British Medical Journal (Clinical Research Ed.). 1986;**293**(6538):6-8. DOI: 10.1136/bmj.293.6538.6

[25] Fuentes B et al. Stroke prevention in patients with type 2 diabetes mellitus or prediabetes. Recommendations of the study Group of Cerebrovascular Diseases of the Spanish Society of Neurology. Neurology. 2021;**36**(4):305-323. DOI: 10.1016/j.nrl.2020.04.030

[26] Rodríguez-Yañez M et al. Prevention of stroke in patients with arterial hypertension: Recommendations of the study Group of Cerebrovascular Diseases of the Spanish Society of Neurology. Neurology. 2021;**36**(6):462-471. DOI: 10.1016/j.nrleng.2020.04.023

[27] Durgan DJ, Ganesh BP, Cope JL, Ajami NJ, Phillips SC, Petrosino JF, et al. Role of the gut microbiome in obstructive sleep apnea-induced hypertension. Hypertension. 2016;**67**:469-474. DOI: 10.1161/hipertensionaha.115.06672

[28] Sánchez Álvarez MJ. Epidemiology and causes of cerebral vascular disease in children. Spanish Journal of Pediatrics. 2017;**73**(Suppl 1):4 ISSN 0034-947X

[29] Spychala MS, Venna VR, Jandzinski M, Doran SJ, Durgan DJ, Ganesh BP, et al. Age-related changes in the gut microbiota influence systemic inflammation and stroke outcome. Annals of Neurology. 2018;**84**(1):23-36. DOI: 10.1002/ana.25250

[30] Osadchiy V, Martin CR, Mayer EA. The gut-brain axis and the microbiome: Mechanisms and clinical implications. Clinical Gastroenterology and Hepatology. 2019;**17**:322-332. DOI: 10.1016/j.cgh.2018.10.002

[31] Postler TS, Ghosh S. Understanding the holobiont: How microbial metabolites affect human health and shape the immune system. Cell Metabolism. 2017;**26**:110-130. DOI: 10.1016/j.cmet.2017.05.008

[32] Zeng X et al. Higher risk of stroke is correlated with increased opportunistic pathogen load and reduced levels of butyrate-producing bacteria in the gut. Frontiers in Cellular and Infection Microbiology. 2019;**9**(4):1-12. DOI: 10.3389/fcimb.2019.00004

[33] Lledós M. New Study Links Gut Microbiota Strains to more Severe Strokes and Poorer Post-Stroke Recovery Was Presented at the 8th European Stroke Organization Conference, Lyon, France: ESOC. May 4-6. 2022. Retrieved from: http://www.recercasantpau.cat/actualitat/un-estudi-relaciona-el-microbioma-intestinal-amb-el-risc-dictus-i-la-seva-evolucio/

[34] Saberi A, Akhondzadeh S, Kazemi S. Infectious agents and stroke: A systematic review. Basic and Clinical Neuroscience. 2021;**12**(4):427-440. DOI: 10.32598/bcn.2021.1324.2

[35] Bonaz B, Bazin T, Pellissier S. The vagus nerve at the interface of the microbiota-gut-brain axis. Frontiers in Neuroscience. 2018;**12**:49. DOI: 10.3389/fnins.2018.00049

[36] Lerner A, Matthias T. Changes in intestinal tight junction permeability associated with industrial food additives explain the rising incidence of autoimmune disease. Autoimmunity Reviews. 2015;**14**(6):479-489. DOI: 10.1016/j.autrev.2015.01.009

[37] Obrenovich M. Leaky gut, leaky brain? Microorganisms. 2018;**6**(4):107. DOI: 10.3390/microorganisms6040107

[38] Pérez-López A et al. Mucosal immunity to pathogenic intestinal bacteria. Nature Reviews Immunology. 2016;**16**(3):135-148. DOI: 10.1038/nri.2015.17

[39] Dokladny K, Zuhl MN, Moseley PL. Intestinal epithelial barrier function and tight junction proteins with heat and exercise. Journal of Applied Physiology. 2016;**120**(6):692-701. DOI: 10.1152/japplphysiol.00536.2015

[40] Chelakkot C, Ghim J, Ryu SH. Mechanisms regulating intestinal barrier integrity and its pathological

implications. Experimental & Molecular Medicine. 2018;**50**(8):1-9. DOI: 10.1038/s12276-018-0126-x

[41] Houlden A. Brain injury induces specific changes in the cecal microbiota of mice through altered autonomic activity and mucoprotein production. Brain, Behavior, and Immunity. 2016;**57**:10-20. DOI: 10.1016/j.bbi.2016.04.003

[42] Cummings, Pomare EW, Branch WJ, Naylos CP, Macfarlane GT. Short-chain fatty acids in the human large intestine, portal, hepatic, and venous blood. Intest. 1987;**28**(10):1221-1227. DOI: 10.1136/gut.28.10.1221

[43] Koh A et al. From dietary fiber to host physiology: Short-chain fatty acids as key bacterial metabolites. Cell. 2016;**165**(6):1332-1345. DOI: 10.1016/j.cell.2016.05.041

[44] Zheng L et al. Microbe-derived butyrate promotes epithelial barrier function through IL-10 receptor-dependent Claudin-2 repression. Journal of Immunology. 2017;**199**(8):2976-2984. DOI: 10.4049/jimmunol.1700105

[45] Dalile B, Van Oudenhove L, Vervliet B, Verbeke K. The role of short-chain fatty acids in microbiota-gut-brain communication. Nature Reviews. Gastroenterology & Hepatology. 2019;**16**(8):461-478. DOI: 10.1038/s41575-019-0157-3

[46] Koeth RA, Wang Z, Levison BS, Buffa JA, Org E, Sheehy BT, et al. Intestinal microbiota metabolism of l-carnitine, a nutrient in red meat, promotes atherosclerosis. Nature Medicine. 2013;**19**:576-585. DOI: 10.1038/nm.3145

[47] Tang WHW, Wang Z, Levison BS, Koeth RA, Britt EB, Fu X, et al. Intestinal microbial metabolism of phosphatidylcholine and cardiovascular risk. The New England Journal of Medicine. 2013;**368**:1575-1584. DOI: 10.1056/NEJMoa1109400

[48] Drexler H. Endothelial dysfunction: Clinical implication. Progress in Cardiovascular Diseases. 1997;**4**:287-324. DOI: 10.1016/s0033-0620(97)80030-8

[49] Zoetendal EG, Smidt H. Endothelial dysfunction: What is the role of the microbiota? Gut. 2018;**67**(2):201-202. DOI: 10.1136/gutjnl-2017-314012

[50] Nordestgaard B, Nielsen L. Atherosclerosis and arterial influx of lipoproteins. Current Opinion in Lipidology. 1994;**5**:252-257. DOI: 10.1097/00041433-199408000-00002

[51] Pillarisetti S. Lipoprotein modulation of subendothelial heparan sulfate proteoglycans (Perlecan) and atherogenicity. Trends in Cardiovascular Medicine. 2000;**10**:60-65. DOI: 10.1016/s1050-1738(00)00048-7

[52] Torres Saura F, Romero Vazquiánez M, Pérez Berbel P, Cotilla de la Rosa E, Diez Ojea B, Arroyo ÚE. New approach to the prevention of stroke in patients with non-valvular fibrillation in hemodialysis: Percutaneous closure of left atrial appendage. Archivos de Cardiología de México. 2020;**90**(1):96-98 Available from: http://www.scielo.org.mx/pdf/acm/v90n1/2604-7063-acm-90-1-96.pdf

[53] Romero Cortés I, Guzmán Morales AG, Islas Ruz FG. Successful thrombolysis in cerebrovascular disease: A case report. Revista de Sanidad Militar. 2018;**72**(5-6):359-362 Available from: http://www.scielo.org.mx/pdf/rsm/v72n5-6/0301-696X-rsm-72-5-6-359.pdf

[54] Rodríguez C, Luque N, Blanco I, Sebastian L, Barberà JA, Peinado VI, et al.

Pulmonary endothelial dysfunction and thrombotic complications in patients with COVID-19. American Journal of Respiratory Cell and Molecular Biology. 2021;**64**(4):407-415. DOI: 10.1165/rcmb.2020-0359PS

[55] Santos García D, Rodríguez Yáñez M, Arias Rivas S, Blanco M. Endothelium-dependent vasodilation in the brachial artery: Use in clinical and experimental neurology. Neurology Journal. 2011;**53**(6):351-353. DOI: 10.33588/rn,5306.2011240

[56] Roncal C, Martínez-Aguilar E, Orbe J, et al. Trimethylamine N-oxide (TMAO) predicts cardiovascular mortality in peripheral arterial disease. Scientific Reports. 2019;**9**:15580 Retrieved from: DOI: 10.1038/s41598-019-52082-z

[57] Orlich MJ, Singh PN, Sabaté J, Jaceldo-Siegl K, Fan J, Knutsen S, et al. Vegetarian dietary patterns and mortality in Adventist health study 2. JAMA Internal Medicine. 2013;**173**(13):1230-1238. DOI: 10.1001/jamainternmed.2013.6473

[58] Bechthold A, Boeing H, et al. Food groups and risk of coronary heart disease, stroke and heart failure: A systematic review and dose-response meta-analysis of prospective studies. Critical Reviews in Food Science and Nutrition. 2019;**59**(7):1071. DOI: 10.1080/10408398.2017.1392288

[59] Strath SJ, Kaminsky LA, Ainsworth ES, et al. Guide to physical activity assessment: Clinical and research applications: A scientific statement from the American Heart Association. Circulation. 2013;**128**:2259-2279. DOI: 10.1161/01.cir.0000435708. 67487.da

[60] Coutts SB, Wein TH, Lindsay MP, Buck B, Cote R, Ellis P, et al. Canadian stroke Best practice recommendations: Secondary prevention of stroke guidelines, update 2014. International Journal of Stroke. 2015;**10**(3):282-291. DOI: 10.1111/ijs.12439

[61] Fuentes B. Antidiabetics in stroke prevention in patients with type 2 diabetes. The neurologist's point of view. Clinical Medicine. 2018;**150**(7):275-281. DOI: 10.1016/j.medcli.2017.09.012

[62] Palacio-Portilla EJ et al. Dyslipidemia and stroke prevention: Recommendations of the cerebrovascular disease study Group of the Spanish Society of neurology. Neurology. 2022;**37**(1):61-72. DOI: 10.1016/j.nrl.2020.07.027

[63] Verma S, Gulati P, Khatter H, et al. Secondary prevention process evaluation protocol using a structured semi-interactive stroke prevention package in the Indian study (SPRINT India). International Journal of Qualitative Methods. 2022; Retrieved from:. DOI: 10.1177/16094069221093139

[64] Kate MP, Verma SJ, Arora D, Sylaja PN, Padma MV, Bhatia R, et al. Systematic development of structured semi-interactive stroke prevention package for secondary stroke prevention. Annals of Indian Academy of Neurology. 2020;**23**(5):681-686. DOI: 10.4103/aian.AIAN_639_19

[65] Khatter H, Pandián JD, Kate M, et al. Statistical analysis plan for secondary prevention using structured semi-interactive stroke prevention package in INDIA (SPRINT INDIA): A randomized controlled trial. Med. International Journal Stroke 2022;**5**:14-20. DOI: 10.1177/1747493019895653

[66] Kamal AK, Jeque Q, Pachá O, et al. A randomized controlled trial of behavioral intervention to improve medication adherence in adult stroke patients with a prescription-tailored short message

service (SMS): SMS4 stroke study. BMC Neurology. 2015;**15**:212. DOI: 10.1186/s12883-015-0471-5

[67] Deng QW et al. Triglyceride to high-density lipoprotein cholesterol ratio predicts worse outcomes after acute ischemic stroke. European Journal of Neurology. 2017;**24**(2):283-291. DOI: 10.1111/ene.13198

[68] Dieplinger B et al. Prognostic value of inflammatory and cardiovascular biomarkers for the prediction of 90-day all-cause mortality after acute ischemic stroke: Results of the Linz stroke unit study. Clinical Chemistry. 2017;**63**(6):1101-1109. DOI: 10.1373/clinchem.2016.269969

[69] Chen XL et al. Serum YKL-40, a prognostic marker in patients with large-artery atherosclerotic stroke. Acta Neurologica Scandinavica. 2017;**136**(2):97-102. DOI: 10.1111/ane.12688

[70] Tiwari P, Dwivedi R, Bansal M, Tripathi M, Dada R. Role of gut microbiota in neurological disorders and its therapeutic significance. Journal of Clinical Medicine. 2023;**12**(4):1650. DOI: 10.3390/jcm12041650

Chapter 7

Key Points of Nursing Care for Patients with Acute Stroke

Yukari Hisaka, Allan Paulo Blaquera, Kensaku Takase and Tetsuya Tanioka

Abstract

In patients with stroke, it has been proven that management by a specialized medical team for stroke treatment for several days immediately after stroke onset significantly reduces mortality, improves return-to-home rates, and positively impacts activities of daily living and quality of life after discharge. This chapter describes the key points of nursing care for patients with acute stroke, which include "Recognition of patients' physical changes," "Prevention of the worsening of acute stroke and related Symptoms," "Reduction of patients' physical distress," "Appropriate management of patients' physical conditions," "Reacquisition of activities of daily living," "Collaboration with rehabilitation therapists," "Reduction of mental and social distress in patients and their families," and "Reduction of the risk of recurrence and requirement of discharge support." These points will have a positive impact on patients with stroke by improving the nurses' competence to practice nursing and enhancing the quality of team care.

Keywords: key points, nursing care, roles, patients with acute stroke, interdisciplinary collaboration

1. Introduction

In patients with stroke, it has been proven that management by a specialized medical team for stroke treatment for several days immediately after stroke onset significantly reduces mortality, improves return-to-home rates, and positively impacts activities of daily living and quality of life after discharge [1–3]. The team includes physicians, nurses, physical therapists, occupational therapists, speech therapists, clinical technologists, pharmacists, nutritionists, and medical social workers. Team care—in which all of these professions work together by contributing their expertise—is highly effective in delivering treatment. Therefore, it is necessary to clarify the role of nurses and key points of nursing care within the stroke support team.

In this chapter, we first report the results of a questionnaire survey of nurses working in SCUs (Stroke Care Units) that provide nursing care to patients with acute stroke in Japan, to determine what kind of nursing care they believe is necessary for patients with acute stroke. Based on this survey, critical nursing care for patients with acute stroke was divided into the following eight categories: "Recognition of patients' physical changes," "Prevention of the worsening of acute stroke and related Symptoms," "Reduction of patients' physical distress," "Appropriate management of patients' physical conditions," "Reacquisition of activities of daily living," "Collaboration with rehabilitation therapists," "Reduction of mental and social distress in patients and their families," and "Reduction of the risk of recurrence and requirement of discharge support."

For each of these eight categories, the key points of nursing care for patients with acute stroke will be explained, taking into account differences by pathological type (cerebral hemorrhage, subarachnoid hemorrhage, cerebral infarction, etc.), severity, site of injury, and time since the onset of stroke.

2. What is nursing care for patients with acute stroke?

The collaboration between neurosurgeons and certified stroke nurses has resulted in the development of 52 key points of nursing care for patients with acute stroke. A web-based survey was conducted among 1040 nurses working in SCUs managing patients with acute stroke in Japan, who responded to each of the 52 points of nursing care using a 5-point scale (5. very important, 4. somewhat important, 3. undecided, 2. not very important, 1. not important at all). The responses of 702 respondents, excluding results with missing values, were included in the analysis. A summary of the subjects is shown in **Table 1**.

Characteristics	Frequency (n)	Percentage (%)
Age		
20–29	312	44.2
30–39	179	25.4
40–49	157	22.2
50 years old and above	58	8.2
Gender		
Female	631	89.4
Male	75	10.6
Years of experience as a nurse		
0–3	148	21.0
4–5	105	14.9
6–10	173	24.5
11–20	167	23.7
21 years and above	113	16.0
Years of experiences taking care for patient with acute stroke		
0–3	333	47.2
4–5	28	4.0
6–10	124	17.6
11–20	145	20.5
21 years and above	76	10.8

Characteristics	Frequency (n)	Percentage (%)
Position		
Nursing manager	67	9.5
Staff nurse	639	90.5
Qualified as a specialist		
Certified nurse specialist	36	5.1
General nurse	670	94.9
Hospital number of beds		
0–99	62	8.8
100–399	297	42.1
400–699	232	32.9
700 beds and above	115	16.3
Number of beds in Stroke Care Unit		
1–9	449	63.6
10 beds and above	257	36.4

Table 1.
Participants' demographic characteristics (N = 706).

Question number and items (N = 706)		Mean	SD
Q1	Should grasp the severity of stroke	4.85	0.37
Q2	Should grasp the treatment progress from the onset of stroke	4.87	0.35
Q3	Should recognize the need for treatment in patients with acute stroke	4.93	0.25
Q4	Should recognize the changes in intracranial hypertension due to stroke	4.94	0.25
Q5	Should recognize the changes in consciousness disorder due to stroke	4.97	0.17
Q6	Should recognize changes in the motor dysfunction due to stroke	4.94	0.23
Q7	Should grasp the changes in sensory dysfunction due to stroke	4.78	0.42
Q8	Should grasp the changes in swallowing dysfunction due to stroke	4.90	0.30
Q9	Should grasp the changes in eye symptoms (pupil diameter, light reflex, eye movement) due to stroke	4.91	0.29
Q10	Should grasp the changes in higher brain dysfunction due to stroke	4.78	0.42
Q11	Should recognize the changes in the general condition of patients with acute stroke	4.94	0.24
Q12	Should grasp the exacerbation risk in patients with acute stroke	4.91	0.28
Q13	Should report changes in the disease state of patients with acute stroke to physicians at the appropriate time	4.97	0.18
Q14	Should provide nursing care to prevent exacerbation of intracranial hypertension in patients with acute stroke	4.92	0.29
Q15	Should provide nursing care to prevent sudden changes in the circulatory dynamics of patients with acute stroke	4.88	0.34
Q16	Should provide nursing care to prevent respiratory complications in patients with acute stroke	4.90	0.31

Question number and items (N = 706)		Mean	SD
Q17	Should ensure that patients with acute stroke receive appropriate treatment from physicians	4.94	0.24
Q18	Should provide nursing care to patients with acute stroke to avoid the risk of secondary complications due to restricted movement	4.85	0.37
Q19	Should provide nursing care to ensure optimal nutrition and fluid intake in patients with acute stroke	4.84	0.39
Q20	Should provide nursing care to patients with acute stroke to avoid the risk of physical injury and to ensure safe medical treatment	4.83	0.40
Q21	Should try to recognize the distress caused to patients with acute stroke as they are unable to communicate to others	4.86	0.37
Q22	Should make attempts to reduce pain due to physical changes caused by a stroke	4.86	0.35
Q23	Should provide nursing care to patients with acute stroke to minimize physical distress through treatment and care	4.85	0.37
Q24	Should defend the human rights of patients with acute stroke who cannot communicate their own desires	4.85	0.41
Q25	Should coordinate with physical therapists, occupational therapists, and speech therapists (hereinafter therapists) in order for patients with acute stroke to be able to receive training/exercise effectively	4.83	0.39
Q26	Should know the details of training/exercises for patients with acute stroke guided by the therapists	4.53	0.59
Q27	Should recognize the maximum physical ability of patients with acute stroke during training/exercise guided by the therapists	4.54	0.61
Q28	Should communicate to therapists about changes in patients with acute stroke that affect their training/exercise	4.76	0.46
Q29	Should facilitate not only therapist-guided training/exercise but also provide training/exercise by nurses	4.46	0.69
Q30	Should provide nursing care to patients with acute stroke to promote their recovery	4.79	0.46
Q31	Should provide nursing care to patients with acute stroke for better sleep and rest	4.82	0.41
Q32	Should provide nursing care to improve consciousness disorder in patients with acute stroke	4.70	0.54
Q33	Should recognize assistance needs and the levels of ADL in patients with acute stroke	4.86	0.35
Q34	Should detect dysfunction-affecting ADL in patients with acute stroke	4.84	0.38
Q35	Should provide nursing care to help patients with acute stroke to regain their ADL	4.82	0.40
Q36	Should help patients with acute stroke to perform ADL by themselves	4.71	0.53
Q37	Should try grasping the mental distress of patients with acute stroke	4.81	0.41
Q38	Should try to recognize the social distress in patients with acute stroke	4.64	0.56
Q39	Should recognize the mental distress in the family of patients with acute stroke	4.75	0.48

Question number and items (N = 706)		**Mean**	**SD**
Q40	Should recognize the need for family support in patients with acute stroke	4.71	0.53
Q41	Should provide nursing care to reduce mental distress in patients with acute stroke	4.79	0.44
Q42	Should provide nursing care to help patients with acute stroke accept their disabilities	4.79	0.45
Q43	Should provide nursing care to help patients with acute stroke that enables them to feel positive	4.74	0.50
Q44	Should provide nursing care for family-related mental distress in patients with acute stroke	4.72	0.51
Q45	Should provide nursing care for the need for family support in patients with acute stroke	4.62	0.60
Q46	Should recognize the medical history and lifestyle risk factors for the onset of stroke in patients with acute stroke	4.85	0.37
Q47	Should explain the risk of recurrence to patients with acute stroke	4.82	0.47
Q48	Should teach patients with acute stroke about lifestyle changes after hospital discharge to avoid the risk of recurrence	4.85	0.40
Q49	Should provide nursing care and guidance to patients with acute stroke (and their families if patient family support is needed in post-discharge life) to avoid the risk of recurrence	4.85	0.41
Q50	Should share the prognosis of patients with acute stroke with other healthcare providers	4.76	0.49
Q51	Should provide nursing care to facilitate the transfer of patients with acute stroke to the hospital	4.77	0.48
Q52	Should provide nursing care to facilitate hospital discharge of patients with acute stroke	4.79	0.47

Table 2.
Perception of the importance of nursing for patients with acute stroke.

Table 2 shows the results of the survey on the perceived needs for the 52 points of nursing care for patients with acute stroke. The mean of responses to all 52 points of nursing care for patients with acute stroke, which were developed independently, was 4.5 or higher out of 5. The items "Should recognize the changes in consciousness disorder due to stroke" and "Should report changes in the disease state of patients with acute stroke to physicians at the appropriate time" averaged 4.97. The items "Should recognize the changes in intracranial hypertension due to stroke," "Should recognize changes in the motor dysfunction due to stroke," "Should recognize the changes in the general condition of patients with acute stroke," and "Should ensure that patients with acute stroke receive appropriate treatment from physicians" had an average value of 4.94. The point of nursing care for these patients with acute stroke was found to be particularly important.

Table 3 shows the names of the eight categories of the exploratory factor analysis. The critical nursing care points included in each category are presented [4]. A conceptual diagram of nursing care for patients with acute stroke is shown in **Figure 1**.

Recognition of patients' physical changes	Should recognize the changes in consciousness disorder due to stroke
	Should report changes in the disease state of patients with acute stroke to physicians at the appropriate time
	Should recognize changes in the motor dysfunction due to stroke
	Should recognize the changes in the general condition of patients with acute stroke
	Should recognize the need for treatment in patients with acute stroke
	Should recognize the changes in intracranial hypertension due to stroke
Prevention of the worsening of acute stroke and related symptoms	Should provide nursing care to prevent sudden changes in the circulatory dynamics of patients with acute stroke
	Should provide nursing care to prevent exacerbation of intracranial hypertension in patients with acute stroke
	Should provide nursing care to prevent respiratory complications in patients with acute stroke
Reduction of patients' physical distress	Should make attempts to reduce pain due to physical changes caused by a stroke
	Should try to recognize the distress caused to patients with acute stroke as they are unable to communicate to others
	Should provide nursing care to patients with acute stroke to minimize physical distress through treatment and care
Appropriate management of patients' physical conditions	Should provide nursing care to patients with acute stroke to avoid the risk of secondary complications due to restricted movement
	Should provide nursing care to ensure optimal nutrition and fluid intake in patients with acute stroke
	Should provide nursing care to patients with acute stroke to avoid the risk of physical injury and to ensure safe medical treatment
	Should ensure that patients with acute stroke receive appropriate treatment from physicians
Reacquisition of activities of daily living	Should recognize assistance needs and the levels of ADL in patients with acute stroke
	Should detect dysfunction-affecting ADL in patients with acute stroke
	Should provide nursing care to help patients with acute stroke to regain their ADL
	Should provide nursing care to patients with acute stroke for better sleep and rest
	Should provide nursing care to improve consciousness disorder in patients with acute stroke
	Should provide nursing care to patients with acute stroke to promote their recovery
	Should help patients with acute stroke to perform ADL by themselves
	Should recognize the medical history and lifestyle risk factors for the onset of stroke in patients with acute stroke
Collaboration with rehabilitation therapists	Should recognize the maximum physical ability of patients with acute stroke during training/exercise guided by the therapists
	Should know the details of training/exercises for patients with acute stroke guided by the therapists
	Should communicate to therapists about changes in patients with acute stroke that affect their training/exercise
	Should facilitate not only therapist-guided training/exercise but also provide training/exercise by nurses
Reduction of mental and social distress in patients and their families	Should provide nursing care for family-related mental distress in patients with acute stroke
	Should recognize the need for family support in patients with acute stroke
	Should provide nursing care for the need for family support in patients with acute stroke
	Should recognize the mental distress in the family of patients with acute stroke
	Should try to recognize the social distress in patients with acute stroke

Reduction of the risk of recurrence and requirement of discharge support	Should teach patients with acute stroke about lifestyle changes after hospital discharge to avoid the risk of recurrence
	Should provide nursing care and guidance to patients with acute stroke (and their families if patient family support is needed in post discharge life) to avoid the risk of recurrence
	Should explain the risk of recurrence to patients with acute stroke
	Should provide nursing care to facilitate the transfer of patients with acute stroke to the hospital
	Should provide nursing care to facilitate hospital discharge of patients with acute stroke
	Should share the prognosis of patients with acute stroke with other healthcare providers

Table 3.
Result of exploratory factor analysis of the perception of the need for nursing for patients with acute stroke scale (excerpt from Ref. [4]).

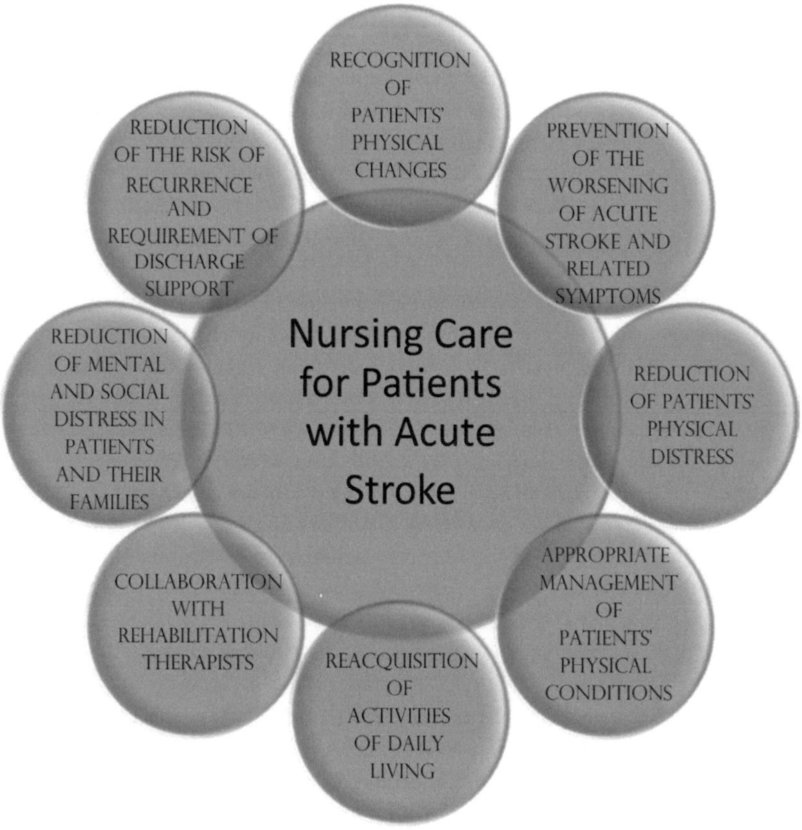

Figure 1.
Conceptual diagram of nursing care for patients with acute stroke.

3. Key points for nursing care for patients with acute stroke

3.1 Recognition of patients' physical changes

"Recognition of patients' physical changes" refers to nursing care to identify changes in general condition and neurological signs due to the onset of stroke and report them to the physician when appropriate.

Patients with cerebral infarction are particularly prone to reinfarction during the acute phase. In addition, when there is extensive cortical damage, cerebral edema may occur, resulting in increased intracranial pressure. Intracranial hemorrhage may also occur following reopening of arterial blood flow in the acute phase with thrombolytic therapy or mechanical thrombus retrieval therapy. Nurses must detect early signs of worsening neurological symptoms or changes in circulatory dynamics due to reinfarction or other causes and report them to the physician. In Japan, periodic evaluation of the degree of consciousness impairment using the Glasgow Coma Scale or the Japan Coma Scale is mandatory. Moreover, the degree of paralysis, sensory deficits, aphasia, and other higher functions, as well as respiratory and circulatory parameters such as blood pressure, respiration, and SaO_2, are often observed over time. The nurses should determine the observation items and timing, taking into consideration the severity of the patient's illness, the number of days since the onset, the site of injury, and the symptoms present. The nurses should also properly evaluate the observations, determine exactly what findings, if any, are likely to worsen the patient's life expectancy or neurological function, and report them to the physician in a timely manner.

Patients with cerebral hemorrhage are at high risk of rebleeding during the acute phase, and rebleeding leads to exacerbation of increased intracranial pressure. In particular, in the case of brainstem and cerebellar hemorrhage, even a relatively small amount of bleeding can be directly life-threatening. When ventricular drainage is used to manage hydrocephalus, physical changes, cerebrospinal fluid pressure, and the amount and nature of drainage fluid should be monitored in combination.

Patients with subarachnoid hemorrhage are at particular risk for rerupture in the time between onset and treatment procedures such as clipping or coil embolization to prevent rupture. Nurses should observe not only for signs of rerupture, but also for elevated blood pressure, pain, and stress, which are risk factors for rerupture. The first two weeks after onset are considered to be the most likely time for stroke due to delayed cerebral vasospasm. During this period, neurological signs should be monitored over time for deterioration and early detection of decreased cerebral blood flow.

The nurses decide what signs should be monitored, taking into consideration the patient's disease type, location of brain injury, severity, treatment, current symptoms, and the number of days since onset and progress. Furthermore, the nurses are responsible for analyzing the assessment data and reporting to the physician if further examination or treatment is needed.

3.2 Prevention of the worsening of acute stroke and related symptoms

"Prevention of the worsening of acute stroke and related symptoms" refers to nursing care that avoids increased intracranial pressure, sudden changes in circulatory dynamics, and respiratory complications.

For the acute stroke patient, the most important nursing care aimed at avoiding critical illness is to prevent cerebral herniation due to intracranial hypertension. The first step is the early detection of signs of intracranial hypertension. Patients at high risk for cerebral edema and rebleeding are also at high risk for cerebral herniation. The nurses should detect signs of intracranial hypertension, such as headache, nausea, and vomiting, changes in the level of consciousness, differences in pupil diameter and size, changes in blood pressure, widening of pulse pressure, bradycardia, changes in breathing patterns, and increased body temperature. When the nurses detect signs of cerebral herniation, they should immediately report it to the physician and assist the physician in quickly alleviating the increased intracranial pressure.

Some reports indicate that raising the head position to 15–30 degrees is effective when intracranial pressure is elevated [5]. The nurses should ensure that the patient is in the most appropriate position, without increasing intracranial pressure, with minimal pain, and with an integrated assessment of the risk of pressure ulcers and prevention of respiratory complications. During this period, it is important to keep the patient comfortable, with appropriate blood pressure control, and to avoid stimulation and minimize physical and emotional stress.

Physiological monitoring has been reported to be effective in patients with acute stroke [6]. Nurses continuously monitor blood pressure and electrocardiograms in patients with acute stroke. Unlike patient management in general diseases, the Japanese Stroke Treatment Guidelines 2021 [7] recommend that hypertension in patients with acute cerebral infarction should not be lowered as much as possible. It states that prudent antihypertensive therapy should be used only when systolic blood pressure > 220 mmHg or diastolic blood pressure > 120 mmHg is sustained. For blood pressure management of patients with acute cerebral hemorrhage, the authors recommend lowering systolic blood pressure to <140 mmHg. Blood pressure control in patients with subarachnoid hemorrhage varies before and after surgical treatment of a ruptured aneurysm and requires strict individualized blood pressure control. After surgery, blood pressure is often maintained and elevated to prevent or treat cerebral vasospasm. The nurses ensure that the appropriate blood pressure for each type of stroke is maintained. The nurses promptly report any deviation from the appropriate blood pressure to the physician or adjusts medications, as previously ordered by the physician, to control the blood pressure. The nurses must also provide assistance with daily activities and aid in encouraging the patient to sit or stand at bedside, while preventing sudden blood pressure changes.

Many patients with acute stroke develop respiratory infections, such as pneumonia resulting in serious illness [8]. Nurses must perform continuous monitoring of respiratory status in patients with acute stroke. It is critical that nurses provide positioning, swallowing training, oral care, and early initiation of physical activity to prevent aspiration and avoid complications such as respiratory infections [9].

3.3 Reduction of patients' physical distress

"Reduction of patients' physical distress" refers to nursing care aimed at identifying and reducing physical distress associated with physical changes and treatment due to stroke.

Stroke patients experience physical pain, such as the inability to move themselves as they did before the onset of the stroke, as well as numbness and pain in the extremities due to sensory disturbance. Other symptoms may include headache, nausea, and vertigo. Headache occurs in 28% of patients with acute stroke [10]. Dizziness is more common in stroke patients with foci in the cerebellum or brainstem. Patients with acute stroke experience these distresses suddenly. These physical distresses further interfere with sleep and rest and increase mental anxiety. Nurses need to alleviate physical pain as much as possible with pharmacologic and nonpharmacologic nursing care. In addition, stroke patients often suffer from aphasia and impaired consciousness [11] and may not be able to communicate their distress to others. Nurses must anticipate what kind of physical pain the patient may experience depending on the location of the brain injury and the pathological condition.

Some treatments, tests, and nursing care provided for patients with acute stroke cause physical distress. For example, frequent and unnecessary monitoring also interfere with sleep. Restricting patient activities for the sake of patient safety can also cause distress. Nurses should provide nursing care with the utmost prudence to ensure patient safety and avoid causing patient distress. Nurses must be keen in addressing physical distress such as sensory disturbance and impaired communication while ensuring comfort and safety.

3.4 Appropriate management of patients' physical conditions

"Appropriate management of patients' physical conditions" refers to nursing care that aims to avoid complications secondary to immobility and to ensure adequate nutrition and fluid intake.

Patients in the acute phase of stroke are often immobile due to impaired consciousness or impaired motor function. Some of their activities are restricted as part of the treatment to prevent sudden intracranial pressure changes. They are prone to disuse syndrome, which is a functional decline in the musculoskeletal, respiratory/circulatory, and psychoneurotic systems. Starting rehabilitation early after the onset of patients with acute stroke can prevent disuse syndrome, but the acute phase of stroke is unstable and requires adequate risk management. Nurses need to observe patients for progression or recurrence of the primary disease condition, detect changes in respiratory and circulatory dynamics, and collaborate with therapists and physicians to safely provide rehabilitation. Therapies may include early initiation of physical activity and self-care training.

Nurses should also implement safety without overloading the patient, such as in the prevention of deep vein thrombosis, aspiration pneumonia, bedsores, and joint contractures, especially when the patient's condition is unstable and aggressive rehabilitation cannot be initiated.

Patients with acute stroke with impaired consciousness, dysphagia, or unstable vital signs are more likely to have poor nutritional status because they are unable to take food and fluids orally [12]. Patients with acute stroke with poor nutritional status are likely to have a poor outcome [13]. Therefore, swallowing evaluation and training should be performed early in the course of illness to initiate oral intake. In Japan, swallowing evaluation and training are often performed by speech-language pathologists. However, to intervene earlier and more frequently, training is also provided by nurses so that it can be performed in accordance with the patient's condition. If oral intake is difficult, enteral nutrition is initiated, such as by inserting nasogastric tubes. Thus, nursing care is focused on enteral feeding management while preventing diarrhea and aspiration in order to maintain good nutritional status and fluid balance.

3.5 Reacquisition of activities of daily living

"Reacquisition of activities of daily living" refers to nursing care aimed at helping patients regain activities of daily living that have declined due to the onset of stroke.

Patients with stroke have diverse sequelae. Three months after stroke, 21.7% of patients had no symptoms at all on the mRS (Modified Rankin Scale) survey, and 48.6% needed some forms of assistance [14]. Rehabilitation and self-care training for patients with acute stroke is effective and recommended to be implemented from early onset [7]. The Agency for Health Care Policy and Research (AHCPR) guidelines also recommend initiating automatic exercises such as turning, sitting posture, and self-care within 24–48 hours of attack, if medically possible [15].

Nurses are responsible for assisting patients with activities of daily living. The nurses should not do all the activities of daily living that the patient cannot perform, but rather assist them to achieve independence. The nurses should also understand the extent to which the patient is unable to perform each activity of daily living, based on an accurate assessment of self-care ability. In Japan, the Barthel Index (BI) or functional independence measure (FIM) are used to assess the activities of daily living of stroke patients. The FIM is applied by nurses in order to evaluate the patient's actual activities of daily living. In some cases, even if there are no motor dysfunctions, the patient may be unable to perform activities of daily living due to fatigue. The patient's maximum capacity for activities of daily living is demonstrated during rehabilitation by the therapist. The nurses compare the patient's maximum ability to perform activities of daily living from actual daily activities, and analyze them to establish the difference. Early initiation of assisting patients in their activities of daily living will have a positive outcome on the subsequent degree of independence.

3.6 Collaboration with rehabilitation therapists

"Collaboration with rehabilitation therapists" refers to nursing care aimed at ensuring that patients with acute stroke effectively receive training from physical therapists, occupational therapists, and speech-language pathologists, as well as nursing care for training by nurses to restore function outside of therapists' training hours.

The nurses' role is to inform the therapist of any changes in the patient that affect training. The nurses inform the rehabilitation therapist of any signs of lesion expansion or recurrence, changes in blood pressure, respiratory status, body temperature, or other general conditions, and distress symptoms such as headache, dizziness, or nausea, and any delirium, anxiety, or decreased motivation. The rehabilitation therapist also collects information in advance and conducts rehabilitation with sufficient risk management.

However, the condition of patients with acute stroke can easily change, and therapy without sufficient understanding of the patient's condition can lead to worsening of the condition or have a negative impact on the patient's physical and mental health. In Japan, the amount of time that therapists spend performing rehabilitation is fixed by health insurance. It is important for patients to decide how to spend their time outside of therapist-led training in order for them to recover their functions and regain their ability to perform activities of daily living. While some training can be performed by the patient themselves, assistance by the nurses is often necessary when it is dangerous or difficult for the patient to perform the tasks independently. The nurses should also consult with the rehabilitation therapist to discuss what kind of training is being performed during rehabilitation and how much and what kind of training should be performed during non-rehabilitation time.

To ensure that the patients receive safe and effective therapy, it is important that nurses and rehabilitation therapists collaborate and communicate regarding any aspect that concerns the patient's present condition and management.

3.7 Reduction of mental and social distress in patients and their families

"Reduction of mental and social distress in patients and their families" refers to nursing care that identifies and supports the mental and social distress of patients and their families.

Stroke is sudden in onset and completely changes a person's life. Patients with acute stroke have difficulty in immediately accepting the sudden changes caused by their condition. The environmental changes of hospitalization and the fear of pain and illness can easily trigger a state of crisis. Furthermore, patients with acute stroke often suffer impaired consciousness and cognitive dysfunction. It takes time for them to understand their own current condition. Post-stroke depression (PSD) constitutes a complication in 33% of patients [16], and many patients have complicated psychiatric symptoms such as post-stroke apathy (PSA) and delirium.

Patients with acute stroke have varying tendencies when it comes to their ability to understand their situation as well as issues with stressors, and communication skills, due to severity of stroke. If the nurses determine that a patient's mental condition requires professional intervention, they should report it to another medical professional. Moreover, PSD, PSA and psychiatric symptoms have been reported to impair activities of daily living and quality of life [17]. Nurses can alleviate the emotional distress of patients with acute stroke, thereby helping them to continue treatment and maintain their motivation to recover.

The sudden onset of stroke can also lead to a state of crisis for the patient's family. Family members of patients in the acute phase of stroke are the voice for the patient who is unable to communicate their wishes, make decisions on behalf of the patient, and support the patient in social roles that the patient is no longer able to fulfill. The nurses' role is to maintain a good mental and social state not only for the patient but this expands also to the family members.

3.8 Reduction of the risk of recurrence and requirement of discharge support

"Reduction of the risk of recurrence and requirement of discharge support" refers to nursing care to coordinate smooth discharge or transfer from the hospital and life guidance after discharge to avoid recurrent strokes.

In Japan, an increasing number of facilities have introduced the Stroke Regional Coordination Pass, which is shared among all healthcare institutions. In these facilities, stroke patients receive treatment, nursing care, and rehabilitation, from the acute phase through the recovery phase to the maintenance phase. The Regional Stroke Coordination Pass allows information to be shared and smoothly coordinated among all medical institutions. This provides stroke patients and their families with sufficient understanding so that the medical team may provide appropriate support. Although the effectiveness of this approach has not been verified in Japan [18], reports show that providing support for early discharge from the acute phase results in reduced long-term dependency and length of hospital stay [19]. Nurses are responsible for planning the transition of stroke patients from the acute phase to a specialized rehabilitation facility or discharge to home.

In a study of stroke recurrence rates in Japan, the 10-year recurrence rates of subarachnoid hemorrhage (SAH), brain hemorrhage, and brain infarction were 70.0%, 55.6%, and 49.7%, respectively [20]. Repeated recurrent strokes are likely to cause new sequelae or to aggravate symptoms, sometimes leading directly to death.

Thus, nurses should understand the differences in risk factors for recurrence according to stroke type. In order to reduce the risk of recurrent stroke after discharge from the hospital, it is important to continue regular checkups and medication [21], blood pressure control [22], smoking cessation [23], dietary management considering hypertension, dyslipidemia, and obesity, as well as engaging in moderate exercise, and observing early detection of signs of recurrent stroke. From the onset of stroke until after discharge, nurses have the critical role of ensuring patients and their families have the capability to manage the burden of stroke in collaboration with the medical team.

4. Conclusion

Nursing care for patients with acute stroke is presented and classified into eight categories. For each category, the author explained the key points of nursing care based on the differences in disease type (cerebral hemorrhage, subarachnoid hemorrhage, cerebral infarction, etc.), severity of stroke, site of injury, and course of stroke. Nursing care for patients with acute stroke is important not only from the physical aspect but also from the mental and social aspects. In addition, nursing care that anticipates not only the current condition but also the future life of the patient is necessary. To this end, we hope that nurses involved with patients with acute stroke will practice the eight categories of nursing care presented in this section. It is important to further accumulate nursing evidence based on practice, improve the quality of nursing care for patients with acute stroke, and provide team care with the aim of minimizing sequelae and promoting patient recovery.

Conflict of interest

The authors declare no conflict of interest.

Author details

Yukari Hisaka[1*], Allan Paulo Blaquera[2], Kensaku Takase[3] and Tetsuya Tanioka[4]

1 Department of Adult Nursing, Gifu University School of Medicine, Japan

2 School of Nursing and Allied Health Sciences, St. Paul University Philippines, Philippines

3 Department of Rehabilitation, Anan Medical Center, Japan

4 Graduate School of Biomedical Sciences, Tokushima University, Japan

*Address all correspondence to: hisaka.yukari.e8@f.gifu-u.ac.jp

References

[1] Indredavik B, Fjaertoft H, Ekeberg G, Løge AD, Mørch B. Benefit of an extended stroke unit service with early supported discharge: A randomized, controlled trial. Stroke. 2000;**31**(12):2989-2994. DOI: 10.1161/01.str.31.12.2989

[2] Stroke Unit Trialists' Collaboration. How do stroke units improve patient outcomes? A collaborative systematic review of the randomized trials. Stroke. 1997;**28**(11):2139-2144. DOI: 10.1161/01.str.28.11.2139

[3] Govan L, Langhorne P, Weir CJ, Stroke Unit Trialists Collaboration. Does the prevention of complications explain the survival benefit of organized inpatient (stroke unit) care?: Further analysis of a systematic review. Stroke. 2007;**38**(9):2536-2540. DOI: 10.1161/STROKEAHA.106.478842

[4] Hisaka Y, Ito H, Yasuhara Y, Takase K, Tanioka T, Locsin R. Nurses' awareness and actual nursing practice situation of stroke care in acute stroke units: A Japanese cross-sectional web-based questionnaire survey. International Journal of Environmental Research and Public Health. 2021;**18**(23):12800. DOI: 10.3390/ijerph182312800

[5] Jauch EC, Saver JL, Adams HP Jr, et al. Guidelines for the early management of patients with acute ischemic stroke: A guideline for healthcare professionals from the American Heart Association/American Stroke Association. Stroke. 2013;**44**(3):870-947. DOI: 10.1161/STR.0b013e318284056a

[6] Ciccone A, Celani MG, Chiaramonte R, Rossi C, Righetti E. Continuous versus intermittent physiological monitoring for acute stroke. Cochrane Database of Systematic Reviews. 2013;**5**:CD008444. DOI: 10.1002/14651858.CD008444.pub2

[7] Miyamoto S, Ogasawara K, Kuroda S, et al. Japan Stroke Society guideline 2021 for the treatment of stroke. International Journal of Stroke. 2022;**17**(9):1039-1049. DOI: 10.1177/17474930221090347

[8] Westendorp WF, Nederkoorn PJ, Vermeij JD, Dijkgraaf MG, van de Beek D. Post-stroke infection: A systematic review and meta-analysis. BMC Neurology. 2011;**11**:110. DOI: 10.1186/1471-2377-11-110

[9] Wagner C, Marchina S, Deveau JA, Frayne C, Sulmonte K, Kumar S. Risk of stroke-associated pneumonia and oral hygiene. Cerebrovascular Diseases. 2016;**41**(1-2):35-39. DOI: 10.1159/000440733

[10] Jørgensen HS, Jespersen HF, Nakayama H, Raaschou HO, Olsen TS. Headache in stroke: The Copenhagen Stroke Study. Neurology. 1994;**44**(10):1793-1797. DOI: 10.1212/wnl.44.10.1793

[11] Japan Stroke Data Bank. Understanding the actual conditions of stroke treatment in Japan using the stroke registry. Report 2021. Available from: https://strokedatabank.ncvc.go.jp/f12kQnRl/wp-content/uploads/27f9c9e8df9c5853644f84616ace7775.pdf

[12] Bouziana SD, Tziomalos K. Malnutrition in patients with acute stroke. Journal of Nutritional Metabolism. 2011;**2011**:167898. DOI: 10.1155/2011/167898

[13] Yoo SH, Kim JS, Kwon SU, Yun SC, Koh JY, Kang DW. Undernutrition as a predictor of poor clinical outcomes in acute ischemic stroke patients. Archives

of Neurology. 2008;**65**(1):39-43. DOI: 10.1001/archneurol.2007.12

[14] Ministry of Health, Labour and Welfare. The Ministry of Health, Labour and Welfare White Paper, 2008 Edition - Facing up to Disabilities and Illnesses, A Society Where All People can Play an Active Role—Prognosis of Stroke Patients (18-65 Years Old). Chart 1-2-6. 2008

[15] Gresham GE, Duncan PW, Stason WB, Adams HP, Adelman AM, Alexander DN, et al. Post Stroke Rehabilitation. Clinical Practice Guideline, No.16. U.s. Department of Health and Human services Public Health Service Agency for Health Care Policy and Research Rockville, Maryland. AHCPR Publication No. 95-0662 May 1995. 1995

[16] Hackett ML, Yapa C, Parag V, Anderson CS. Frequency of depression after stroke: A systematic review of observational studies. Stroke. 2005;**36**(6):1330-1340. DOI: 10.1161/01.STR.0000165928.19135.35

[17] Stangeland H, Orgeta V, Bell V. Poststroke psychosis: A systematic review. Journal of Neurology, Neurosurgery, and Psychiatry. 2018;**89**(8):879-885. DOI: 10.1136/jnnp-2017-317,327

[18] Honda S, Tokunaga M, Watanabe S, et al. Survey of stroke types in acute hospitals and Kaifukuki rehabilitation wards: Nine years of Kumamoto Stroke Liaison Critical Pathway data. Japanese Journal of Stroke. 2018;**40**:343-349. DOI: 10.3995/jstroke.10569

[19] Langhorne P, Baylan S. Early supported discharge trialists. Early supported discharge services for people with acute stroke. Review Cochrane Database System Review. 2017;7:7

[20] Hata J, Tanizaki Y, Kiyohara Y, et al. Ten year recurrence after first ever stroke in a Japanese community: The Hisayama study. Journal of Neurology, Neurosurgery, and Psychiatry. 2005;**76**(3):368-372. DOI: 10.1136/jnnp.2004.038166

[21] Glader EL, Sjölander M, Eriksson M, Lundberg M. Persistent use of secondary preventive drugs declines rapidly during the first 2 years after stroke. Stroke. 2010;**41**(2):397-401. DOI: 10.1161/STROKEAHA.109.566950

[22] Katsanos AH, Filippatou A, Manios E, et al. Blood pressure reduction and secondary stroke prevention: A systematic review and metaregression analysis of randomized clinical trials. Hypertension. 2017;**69**(1):171-179. DOI: 10.1161/HYPERTENSIONAHA.116.08485

[23] Pan B, Jin X, Jun L, Qiu S, Zheng Q, Pan M. The relationship between smoking and stroke: A meta-analysis. Medicine (Baltimore). 2019;**98**(12):e14872. DOI: 10.1097/MD.0000000000014872

Chapter 8

Quantifying Spasticity: A Review

Kristjana Ósk Kristinsdóttir, Samuel Ruipérez-Campillo and Þórður Helgason

Abstract

A precise method to measure spasticity is fundamental in improving the quality of life of spastic patients. The measurement methods that exist for spasticity have long been considered scarce and inadequate, which can partly be explained by a lack of consensus in the definition of spasticity. Spasticity quantification methods can be roughly classified according to whether they are based on neurophysiological or biomechanical mechanisms, clinical scales, or imaging techniques. This article reviews methods from all classes and further discusses instrumentation, dimensionality, and EMG onset detection methods. The objective of this article is to provide a review on spasticity measurement methods used to this day in an effort to contribute to the advancement of both the quantification and treatment of spasticity.

Keywords: spasticity, Ashworth scale, Tardieu scale, Wartenberg pendulum test, stretch reflex, electromyography

1. Introduction

Spasticity is a motor impairment present in patients with various neurological disorders, including stroke [1], spinal cord injury (SCI) [2], cerebral palsy (CP) [3], and multiple sclerosis (MS) [4]. It is characterized by the hypersensitivity of the stretch reflex, but its complete mechanisms are poorly understood [5]. Spasticity affects the mobility, and therefore quality of life of those living with it. A precise method to quantify spasticity is, thus, fundamental for early intervention and correct treatment to optimize recovery outcomes and to evaluate other conditions and diseases.

In 1980, Lance proposed a definition of spasticity that, to this day, has been the most prominent one. Lance's definition states that spasticity is "a motor disorder characterized by a velocity-dependent increase in tonic stretch reflexes with exaggerated tendon jerks, resulting from hyperexcitability of the stretch reflex, as one component of the upper motor neuron syndrome" [6]. However, Lance's definition only describes spasticity during passive movement and does not take its effects during voluntary activity into account. As a result, Young proposed a refined definition of spasticity that is independent of the type of movement. Young's definition states that spasticity is "a motor disorder characterized by velocity-dependent increase in tonic stretch reflexes that result from abnormal intraspinal processing of primary afferent input" [7]. More definitions of spasticity have been proposed [8, 9], but there is a lack of consensus regarding which one to use [10–12], which highlights the complexity of the pathology.

Mechanisms that contribute to the development of spasticity include changes in reflex arcs that affect motor neurons' excitability and the changes of motor neurons' internal features [13]. These changes cause a loss of control between the brain and spinal cord, which results in a lack of inhibition of the stretch reflex. In a healthy individual, a stretch of the muscle will activate muscle spindles, which send sensory inputs to the spinal cord through Ia afferent fibers. There, a-motoneurons are activated and send signals to the muscle from which the sensory input arose, causing it to contract. In spasticity, a reduction or a complete loss of the inhibitory effects of the dorsal reticulospinal tract on the a-motoneurons in the spinal cord leads to excessive muscle activation [1, 14], but spasticity can also be caused by increased excitation in motor tracts originating in the brain stem and increased action potentials in sensory neurons [15]. As previously mentioned, the velocity dependence of spasticity has been contributed to changes in the Ia afferent pathway or a change in the gain or threshold of the stretch reflex. Additionally, some studies have suggested a position dependence of spasticity, which might be a result of changes in the gain or threshold of the Ia and group II muscle spindle afferent fibers [10], as well as the viscoelastic properties of the passive tissue of a joint [16].

Since the onset of the neural lesion in spastic CP occurs in an underdeveloped nervous system, there is a differentiation between stroke and SCI patients in the mechanism of spasticity. Carr et al. [17] presented evidence that the descending pathways in patients with perinatal brain injury are subject to reorganization, which leads to a persistence of abnormal reflexes and automatic responses that are not visible in stroke and SCI patients [18]. Further, Willerslev-Olsen et al. [19] reported that passive muscle properties are changed in children as young as three years of age.

Spasticity does not only consist of neurogenic resistance but can also involve complex changes in muscular systems, leading to non-neurogenic resistance [1, 12, 20, 21]. These changes, which may include alterations in muscle fiber size and length along with modifications in fiber type distributions, are not accounted for in Lance's definition [6, 22]. The concentrations of fatigue-resistant muscle fibers in spastic muscle have been reported to exceed that of healthy muscle and changes in mechanical and morphological properties of intra- and extracellular materials may also contribute to spasticity [23–27]. Consequently, it is logical that spasticity assessment consists of both neurophysiological and biomechanical measurements [28]. Moreover, it is important to be able to clinically distinguish neurogenic and non-neurogenic resistance [19] and individually identify which one has a greater contribution to spasticity. Thereby, treatment plans can be constructed based on the profile of components, those with greater neurogenic components may be better suited for a therapy reducing the spinal stretch reflex, while those with a greater non-neurogenic component might benefit from stretch and exercise [20].

As suggested by the preceding discussion, the measurement of spasticity can be extremely complicated. Spasticity has intrinsic fluctuations, whereas it is both time [29, 30] and context-dependent [22]. Therefore, a measurement of the severity of spasticity of an individual can yield completely different results based on, for example, the time of day and physical and emotional state of the subject. The ideal spasticity measurement method should be sensitive to spasticity, clinically feasible, and have high reliability and reproducibility. Further, the elicitation of spasticity has to be standardized. The clinical feasibility of a measurement tool depends on the time required to administer the test, interpret the results, and analyze them. Other factors that come into play include its portability, cost and the need for specialized equipment and training [31]. The objective of this article is to review articles on spasticity measurement methods, and thus provide a platform to advance both the quantification and treatment of spasticity.

2. Clinical scales

As of today, various proposals have been made on how to quantify spasticity. Rating scales, such as the Ashworth and Tardieu scales, are the most prevalent methods for clinical assessment of spasticity, but they are not impeccable. In this section, measurement of spasticity using clinical scales will be discussed. For a clear understanding of this section, a summary of the clinical scales is depicted in **Table 1**. The testing procedure is based on initiating a brisk dorsiflexion movement of the relaxed ankle, activating the monosynaptic stretch reflex pathway [32]. The original Ashworth scale (AS) has been refined [33] to the modified Ashworth Scale (MAS) [34] and the modified modified Ashworth scale (MMAS) [35] to ensure better sensitivity. In fact, those methods have faced controversy, whereas they are dependent upon the subjective interpretation of the examiner and thus suffer from poor inter-rater reliability [39]. The Ashworth scales measure the resistance of a spastic limb during passive soft-tissue stretching and do not take in to account different stretch velocities. Therefore, the AS and MAS cannot indicate whether the resistance is due to a hyperactive stretch reflex or an increase in the viscoelastic properties of other tissues surrounding the joint [12, 36, 40], although MAS has been shown to correlate with surface electromyography (sEMG) stretch response activity [41]. Moreover, a clustering of the values in the mid-range of the MAS has been reported, that is the extreme values are scarce [42] and the MAS has been demonstrated to be more closely related to the passive stiffness of the joint than to joint spasticity [40, 43]. The stiffness of a joint is defined as its resistance to passive movement and indicates the increment in force of the muscles in response to a change in length [44]. In fact, spasticity is only one of many factors that can alter the resistance to passive movement of a joint [45].

Clinical Scale	Procedure	Year	Reference
AS	Patient in supine position. Test a muscle that flexes/extends a joint: place the joint in a maximally flexed/extended position and move to a position of maximal extension/flexion over 1 second.	1964	[32]
MAS		1999	[33, 34]
MMAS		2006	[35]
TS	Muscle's response to different stretch velocities and by determining the spasticity angle. Procedure: The patient will be in testing position according to the muscle to be tested. The stretching velocities of V1 and V3 will be applied to measure R2 and R1, respectively. The quality of muscle reaction will be graded at the stretching velocity of V3 as well. The difference between R2 and R1 will be the measure of the dynamic component of spasticity. V1: As slow as possible. V2: Speed of the limb segment falling – gravitational pull. V3. Fast rate - > gravitational pull. R1: Angle of catch seen at Velocity V2 or V3 R2: Full range of motion achieved when muscle is at rest and tested at V1 velocity	1954	[36]
MTS		1969	[37]
ASAS	The slow passive movement is assessed prior to the fast passive movement, which aids in excluding the nonneural components. Scoring criteria of the ASAS are mutually exclusive, ensuring that each muscle group only fits into one category.	2016	[38]

Table 1.
Summary of the clinical scales and their date and main description for the procedure.

On the other hand, the TS and MTS compare the response of the muscle to passive movement at both slow and fast speeds allowing them to address the velocity-dependent aspect of spasticity and differentiate between neural and soft tissue components of muscle resistance [36, 37]. MTS has been demonstrated to have higher reliability than MAS [32, 39] and is recommended by two international consensus statements as it coordinates with Lance's definition of spasticity [46, 47]. Several parameters obtained from the TS and MTS are used to grade the severity of spasticity. These parameters include the angle of catch (AOC), the type of muscle reaction (X value), and the spasticity angle, which is the difference in the range of motion (ROM) of the joint at different speeds [32].

Although the MTS has been widely used and accepted, there is still a demand for a simple and portable clinical tool that has high levels of validity and reliability. Also, the application of the most frequently used clinical scales can be lengthy, making their usefulness in clinical, and especially pediatric settings insufficient. In this respect, Love et al. [38] extracted the best features from the TS and MTS to create a new clinical scale, the Australian Spasticity Assessment Scale (ASAS). The ASAS has a simple test procedure. Where the slow passive movement is assessed prior to the fast passive movement, which aids in excluding the nonneural components. The scoring criteria of the ASAS are mutually exclusive, ensuring that each muscle group only fits into one category. The inter-rater reliability of the ASAS proved to be greater than that of the most prevalent clinical scales, but it faces a limitation in the distribution of scores, whereas there are many scores of the lowest level but few scores of the highest level [38]. An illustrative summary of the clinical scales is depicted in **Table 1** for clarity. Scholtes et al. [48] created the spasticity test (SPAT) for the same purpose. However, the SPAT is merely a simplification of the TS and does not adopt features from the MTS. The SPAT is clinically feasible considering that its implementation takes a maximum of 15 minutes, and it has excellent intra-rater reliability [48].

3. Instrumental assessment methods

Obtaining a reliable outcome from the MTS is dependent upon the accuracy of the evaluation of the joint angle and angular velocity (see **Table 2**). Therefore, the addition of an instrumented or sensor-based assessment to the clinical scales should significantly improve their accuracy. Banky et al. utilized a Microsoft Kinect 3D camera and a smartphone in order to determine the joint start angle, end angle, total range of motion (ROM), and peak angle velocity while carrying out the MTS. Their results demonstrated a good accuracy compared to a criterion-standard 3D motion analysis system, which establishes that low-cost, accessible technology can be successfully used in instrumented spasticity tests [49]. In a study that investigated the accuracy of AOC measurements using goniometry, van den Noort et al. concluded that the inevitable repositioning of joints after the event of a catch decreases the precision and accuracy of the measurement. Instead of using goniometers, they suggested the use of inertial sensors [16]. Subsequently, Paulis et al. compared the reliability of TS measurements when using goniometers and inertial sensors. They confirmed the findings of van den Noort et al., recommending inertial sensors instead of goniometers to obtain more accurate results [37].

Instrumented tests can be classified according to whether the limb is moved around the joint by an operator [50, 51] or a mechatronic device [52] and the type of biological signals being measured. The added value of instrumented measurements is

Grade	MTT	MT	AS	MAS	MMAS
0	No resistance throughout the course of the passive movement.	No increase in muscle tone.	No increase in muscle tone.	No increase in muscle tone.	No increase in muscle tone.
1	Slight resistance throughout the course of the passive movement, with no clear catch at precise angle.	Slight increase in muscle tone, manifested by a catch and release or by minimal resistance at the end of the range of motion when the affected part(s) is moved in flexion or extension.	Slight increase in muscle tone, manifested by a catch when the limb is moved in flexion or extension.	Slight increase in muscle tone, manifested by a catch and release.	Slight increase in muscle tone, manifested by a catch and release.
1+	—	—	—	Slight increase in muscle tone, manifested by a catch, followed by minimal resistance.	—
2	Clear catch at precise angle, interrupting the passive movement, followed by release.	Marked increase in muscle tone, manifested by a catch in the middle range and resistance throughout the remainder of the range of motion, but affected part (s) easily moved.	More marked increased in muscle tone, but limb easily flexed.	More marked increased in muscle tone through most of the ROM, but affects part(s) easily moved.	Slight increase in muscle tone, manifested by a catch, followed by minimal resistance.
3	Fatigable clonus (10 s when maintaining pressure) occurring at precise angle.	Considerable increase in muscle tone, passive movement difficult.	Considerable increase in muscle tone, passive movement difficult.	Considerable increase in muscle tone, passive movement difficult.	More marked increased in muscle tone through most of the ROM, but affects part(s) easily moved.
4	Infatigable clonus (10 s when maintaining pressure) occurring at precise angle.	Affected part(s) rigid in flexion or extension.	Affected part(s) rigid in flexion or extension.	Affected part(st) regid in flexion or extension.	Considerable increase in muscle tone, passive movement difficult.
5	—	—	—	—	Affected part(s) rigid in flexion or extension.

Table 2.
Overview of evaluation criteria for clinical scales in spasticity quantification.

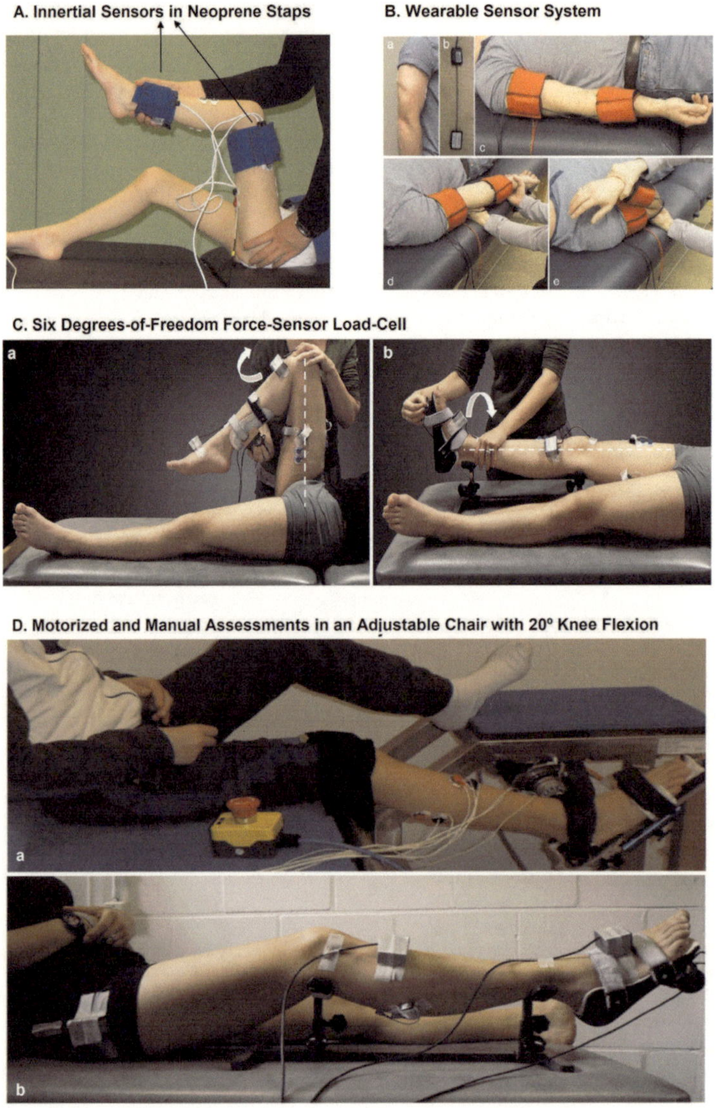

Figure 1.

Illustration of setups and mechanisms in the context of instrumental assessment methods for spasticity. ***A:*** *Spasticity assessment test designed for a child with cerebral palsy to assess spasticity using inertial sensors. The knee joint is in ref. position, with the inertial sensors in the proximal and distant segment. The goniometer does not appear in the figure (extracted over modified figures in [16])* ***B:*** *Assessment of elbow spasticity during passive stretch reflect through the use of a wearable sensor system. (B.a) illustration of the placement of the electrodes on the triceps and bices with two-channel EGM system. (B.b) fiber-optic goniometer. (B.c) wearable sensory system in the arm. (B.d) stretch-reflex test perform by a therapist with limb in extension and (B.e) limb in flexion (extracted over modified figures in [50]).* ***C:*** *Six degrees-of-freedom force-sensor load-cell to measure spasticity. (C.a) the white arrows indicate the direction of the stretch for the medial hamstrings, ensuring that the upper leg is maintained at 90° hip flexion. (C.b) white arrows measure the stretch of the gastrocnemius with a predefined knee angle measured with a calibration trial. Note that for both (C.a) and (C.b), the muscle activity was measured with surface EGM, joint-range characteristics with inertial measurement units, and torque with a force-sensor attached to either a shank orthosis on the posterior aspect of the lower leg or a foot (extracted over modified figures in [51]).* ***D:*** *Study for the evaluation of motorized and manual assessments of spasticity. Participants were seated with 70° hip flexion to limit posture-dependent reflex activity, and 20° knee flexion to allow for small knee contractures and to measure spasticity simultaneously in both the gastrocnemius medialis and soleus muscles. Participants were seated in an adjustable chair for the assessment with motorized (D.a) and on an examination table with a semi-inclined back and the lower leg on a stand for manual assessment (D.b) (extracted over modified figures in [53]).*

their facilitation in quantifying the muscle response, but they also aid in standardizing the imposed movement of a limb by providing feedback [53]. Isokinetic dynamometers have frequently been used in laboratory conditions, but their high cost and limited clinical feasibility decrease their value as spasticity measurement devices [31, 54]. Sloot et al. compared the use of manual and motorized instrumented measurements when assessing the joint resistance in children with CP. The additional value of motorized instrumented tests is that they permit more control in the imposed movement. Their results demonstrated different muscle responses for manual and motorized tests, although the maximum velocity was equal. It was hypothesized that the different muscle responses were due to different movement profiles and that the profile of the manual instrumented test was more similar to that of walking. Furthermore, Sloot et al. suggested that movement profiles of instrumented measurements should match functional tasks, such as walking (**Figure 1**) [53].

4. Biomechanical methods

Biomechanical methods to measure spasticity are concentrated on the resistance to passive movement (RTPM) of a joint. Generally, an effort is made to quantify the forces and torque generated during passive movement using dynamometers [16]. The system designed by Pandyan et al. [55] is a good illustration of the class of biomechanical spasticity measurement methods. The system consists of a force transducer and a flexible electrogoniometer and is designed in order to take simultaneous measurements of applied force and passive range of movement. The RTPM is then calculated as the slope of the graph of these two parameters, yielding a measure with units of Newtons per degrees (N/deg). Kumar et al. used the system developed by Pandyan et al. to assess the validity of MAS by comparing it to the RTPM, applied force, angular displacement, mean velocity, passive range of motion (PROM), and time required for the passive movement. Their results suggested that the MAS is not a valid measure of RTPM or spasticity [56]. A great advantage of the system developed by Pandyan et al. is that it can both be used in bed-bound and fully mobile patients. On the other hand, the system may be susceptible to artifacts as a result of motion at the interface of the apparatus and participant's forearm, which is due to the fact that the clinician is moving the apparatus and not the forearm directly [55]. Lindberg et al. produced a mechanical measurement device and a model that can differentiate the neural component of spasticity from the mechanical components by only monitoring the force during slow and fast passive movements [20]. They found that the neural component was dominating in the majority of the subjects included, who were all chronic stroke patients. They also divided the nonneural components into three categories based on whether they were viscous, elastic, or inertial. The device designed by Lindberg et al., which is devoted to measuring finger and wrist spasticity, has been shown to have higher reliability than the MAS [22]. Active or voluntary movement can also be used to biomechanically quantify spasticity. Wang et al. [57] used a few biomechanical parameters derived from the maximal isometric voluntary contraction of the elbow flexors to quantify spasticity. These parameters included the peak reflex torque (Tp [Nm]), which represented the muscle strength and the keep time of the peak torque (Tk [s]) which indicated the muscle endurance and was defined as the duration for which the muscle strength was maintained above 80% of the maximum torque. Furthermore, the rise time of the peak torque (Tr [s]) which signified the muscle power was defined as the time span between

10% and 80% of the maximum torque. Their results demonstrated that Tk had the best correlation to the severity of spasticity [57].

The Wartenberg pendulum test is based on oscillatory resistance characteristics of the lower limbs and can, therefore, be classified as a biomechanical measurement method. The pendulum test was introduced in the 1950s as a method of assessing spasticity in the clinical setting [58] and has proven to be sensitive to the presence and severity of spasticity [59, 60]. The test itself is based on letting the lower leg swing freely under the influence of gravity while recording joint kinematics. The pendulum test is most commonly used to quantify extensor spasticity, but the presence of flexor spasticity does not affect the results [61]. Initially, six or seven swings around the knee joint were considered normal. A decrease in the time of the leg swing or the number of oscillations was considered to be an indication of upper motor neuron involvement, whereas a prolonged swinging of the knee was contributed to lower motor neuron involvement [58]. However, in 1984, Bajd and Vodovnik [30] instrumented the pendulum test and derived the relaxation indices (R1 and R2) from it. The relaxation indices, which are defined as ratios of the amplitudes of different parts of the leg swing, have been shown to have high variability and low repeatability [60]. Therefore, various new parameters, such as the maximum velocity and acceleration [59, 60, 62], area under the pendulum curve [63], and frequency [62], have been extracted from the pendulum test and used to quantify spasticity. White et al. performed three-dimensional pendulum test analysis on children with CP, as well as able-bodied children. Overall, they extracted 13 parameters from the pendulum test and concluded that the integral of the sagittal plane motion curve [°s] is a better measure of spasticity than the relaxation indices. The integral of the sagittal plane is defined as area under the kinematic curve as a sum of degrees of knee motion by time component and a smaller number indicates more severe spasticity. In fact, White et al. also reported that three-dimensional analysis may be unnecessary since the motion in the frontal and transverse planes is relatively small during the test. They concluded that the pendulum test measures the combined effect of the reflex component of spasticity, chronic changes in musculotendinous tissues, and the muscle tone [62]. Cutting-edge technology has also proved to be useful in the implementation of the pendulum test. Bohannon et al. [63] used a magnetic position tracking system to better characterize the joint kinematics during the testing procedure, and Yeh et al. [64] used empirical mode decomposition along with phase-amplitude coupling analysis between sEMG and joint movement to quantify spasticity. A prominent challenge in the application of the pendulum test is insufficient data on the interaction between muscle activity and joint kinematics due to limited swinging of severely spastic patients. However, the nonlinear parameters described by Yeh et al. [64] overcome that challenge.

Myotonometry is a new technique that measures the stiffness of muscle tissue, and therefore provides an objective assessment of spasticity [65]. The stiffness is measured by pushing a probe onto a muscle and the underlying tissue and quantifying tissue displacement with respect to perpendicular compression force [66, 67]. Measurements can both be performed at rest and during muscle contraction and have been shown to correlate with the RMS of surface electromyography (sEMG) data [67]. Myotonometry benefits from fast data acquisition, easy analysis procedures, and high intra- and inter-rater reliabilities [68].

The concept of spastic catch or the angle of catch (AOC), which was initially described by Tardieu, Shentoub and Delaru [69], has been further researched and refined over the years. The AOC is nowadays most commonly assessed using the MTS and is defined as the angle at which a sudden increase of resistance is felt as a reaction to fast passive stretch. Wu et al. [70] developed an evaluation device consisting of a torque sensor to measure the joint torque and a potentiometer to measure the joint angle. Consequently, they were able to analyze four parameters, namely the position, torque, velocity and torque rate, and investigate their relationship to the AOC. They determined that the AOC is related to the velocity of the joint and further hypothesized that this velocity dependence might be due to a position dependence. Moreover, they discovered that the peak of torque change rate should be used as an indicator of the catch angle [42, 70]. Bar-On et al. [71] investigated the role of joint velocity and torque signals in the measurement of the catch angle. The torque was measured using force sensors at the medial hamstrings and gastrocnemius. They constructed three different definitions of the AOC, the first one based on the position of the maximum deceleration, the second one based on the position of the maximum rate of change of the torque, and the third one based on the angular position corresponding to the first local minimum of power after a local maximum of power. The power was defined as the product of the angular velocity and torque, and consequently, the third definition combines both signals. They found that all the AOC definitions were reliable, although the third definition was the best one. This is due to the fact that the individual signals of velocity and torque were lacking correlation so their integration proved to be the most advantageous. A summary of the most relevant biomechanical methods described in this section is displayed in **Table 3**, organized by relevant author/s, brief description, and main advantages and limitations in a nutshell.

Author	Method/Device	Description/ Conclusions	Advantages	Limitations
Pandyan et al.	Force transducer and flexible electrogoniometer	Take simultaneous measurements of applied force and passive range of movement and calculate RTPM as the slope of the graph of these two parameters.	Can be used in bed-bound and fully mobile patients.	Susceptible to artifacts due to motion at the interface of the apparatus and participant's forearm.
Lindberg et al.	Mechanical measurement device and model	Differentiate neural component of spasticity from mechanical components by monitoring force during slow and fast passive movements.	High reliability.	Limited to finger and wrist spasticity.
Wang et al.	Maximal isometric voluntary contraction of elbow flexors	Quantify spasticity using peak reflex torque, keep time of peak torque, and rise time of peak torque.	Good correlation to severity of spasticity.	Limited to elbow spasticity.
Wartenberg	Wartenberg Pendulum test	Assess spasticity based on oscillatory resistance characteristics of lower limbs.	Sensitive to presence and severity of spasticity	Relatively low repeatability and high variability of relaxation indices.
Bajd and Vodovnik et al.	Relaxation indices (R1 and R2) (on Wartenberg Pendulum Test)	Define relaxation indices as the ratios of amplitudes of different	Objective and quantitative measure.	High variability and low repeatability.

Author	Method/Device	Description/ Conclusions	Advantages	Limitations
		parts of the leg swing, in the pendulum test.		
Fowler et al., Syczewska et al., Bohannon et al., White et al.	Various parameters extracted from the pendulum test (e.g. maximum velocity and acceleration, area under the pendulum curve, frequency).	Extraction of 13 parameters from the pendulum test and used the integral of the sagittal plane motion curve [°s] as a better measure of spasticity than the relaxation indices.	Evaluation of the pendulum test.	Relatively low repeatability and high variability of relaxation indices.
Leonard et al.	Myotonometry	Measures stiffness of muscle tissue using a probe and quantifying tissue displacement with respect to perpendicular compression force. Can be performed at rest and during muscle contraction. Correlates with RMS of sEMG data. High intra- and inter-rater reliabilities.	Fast data acquisition, easy analysis procedures. Provides objective assessment of spasticity.	May be limited by variations in muscle temperature, probe position, and tissue thickness.
Tardieu, Shentoub, and Delaru	Angle of catch (AOC)	Assessed using the MTS as the angle at which a sudden increase of resistance is felt as a reaction to fast passive stretch. Can be measured using torque and potentiometer sensors to analyze position, torque, velocity, and torque rate. Peak of torque change rate can be used as an indicator of the catch angle.	Can be used to determine optimal treatment strategies. Provides information on position, torque, velocity, and torque rate.	May be affected by variations in joint velocity and torque signals. May be limited by lack of correlation between velocity and torque signals.

Table 3.
Summary of the biomechanical methods to assess spasticity and their description, advantages, and limitations in a nutshell.

5. Neurophysiological methods

The AOC can be regarded as a biomechanical method, whereas it is focused on the resistance felt in a joint. However, with the addition of sEMG, the similar mechanisms of the stretch reflex can be analyzed [16]. The stretch reflex (SR) is defined as a sudden increase in muscle activity during a fast passive stretch of a joint and is of a neurophysiological origin. Based on the fact that the muscle activity onset of the stretch reflex precedes the resistance felt in the AOC measurements, van den Noort et al. [16] contemplated that the muscle activity due to a hyperactive stretch reflex is the cause of the catch felt in fast passive stretching. The stretch reflex can be characterized by the threshold at which it is elicited or the reflex gain [72], which is defined as the change in number of motoneurons recruited per change in muscle length. The stretch reflex threshold has been demonstrated to provide a better measure of spasticity than the gain [18, 73–75], and Lance's definition [6] indeed suggests that the stretch reflex threshold should be the core of spasticity measurements. The concept of the SR threshold is based on the lambda model of motor control, which was formulated by Feldman et al. [76]. The lambda model, also called the equilibrium point hypothesis states that within a certain threshold (defined as l- to l+) the stretch reflex can be regulated, whereas in that range the central nervous system can control the joint angle and muscle torque appropriately. In non-spastic subjects, these thresholds lie outside the biomechanical range of joints but with the onset of neurological damage to the descending pathways, one limit of the threshold range might be shifted so that it is located within the biomechanical range and the patient has no ability to shift it. This leads to the hypersensitivity of the stretch reflex and the premature muscle contractions that are characteristic for spasticity [18, 73, 74].

Various different mechanisms, definitions, and methods to measure this threshold have surfaced. The quantification of the stretch reflex threshold is often carried out using either force coordinates or the latency at which muscle activity is elicited following a stretch [77]. However, following the development of the lambda model of motor control, the thresholds are generally expressed in velocity and angular coordinates [52, 78]. As a consequence of the velocity-dependent aspect of spasticity, dissimilar SR thresholds are encountered at different velocities. These are the dynamic SR thresholds (DSRT), and the slope of their regression line is defined as the sensitivity of the stretch reflex (). A positive value is indicative of a damping response to passive stretch dependent on velocity, while a negative value indicates an anti-damping response. Increased sensitivity to the stretch reflex can be explained by reduced presynaptic inhibition of Ia primary fiber afferent inputs but might also be the result of deficits in dynamic fusimotor control of muscle spindle afferent discharges [79]. The tonic SR threshold (TSRT), which is generally defined as the muscle length at which motoneuronal recruitment begins, can be determined by the extrapolation of the regression line of the dynamic SR thresholds to a zero velocity but can also be estimated using quasi-static stretches of the muscle. The two methods have been shown to yield similar results [80]. The TSRT can be viewed as the angle below which the joint can be statically positioned without interference from unwanted muscle contraction [18, 52] or the excitability of motoneurons at zero velocity. When the TSRT lies within the biomechanical range of motion of a joint, spasticity is considered to be present. Additionally, the TSRT is inversely proportional to the severity of spasticity, namely the lower the TSRT, the more severe the spasticity is considered [52]. The sensitivity of the stretch reflex () has been shown to positively correlate with the TSRT in spastic muscles [18, 52].

Musampa et al. [81] used the concept of the SR threshold to establish the approach of spatial spasticity zones, which are the configurations of a joint in which spasticity is present. They then characterized each threshold borderline by its position in joint space and its shape and confirmed a reduction in the range of regulation of the stretch reflex in spastic patients. At last, they found abnormal muscle activation patterns of agonist and antagonist muscles of the whole shoulder joint space during stretch. This finding was also described by Jobin and Levin [18] who studied the SR threshold in children with CP. Germanotta et al. [52] further investigated the stretch reflex in children with CP using a robotic device to impose muscle responses at controlled velocities and compared it to that of typically developing children. Their results demonstrate that using the TSRT approach to measure spasticity of the plantarflexors of the ankle joint in children with CP is indeed feasible and that the addition of a mechatronic instrument is advantageous. Moreover, they confirmed the findings of Pisano et al. who hypothesized that involuntary muscle responses could also be elicited in healthy individuals [44, 82].

Calota et al. [52] developed the montreal spasticity measure (MSM), a portable device that exploits the concept of the stretch reflex. The MSM, which consists of a single-channel EMG, an electrogoniometer, and a laptop computer, measures the DSRT, while a clinician induces a passive stretch at different velocities. This enables a greater variability of input stretch velocities, thereby achieving a more reliable estimate of the TSRT. A moderate reliability for the MSM was reported, but there was no correlation between the TSRT values reported and the MAS scores. This finding, which is relatively prevalent for neurophysiological parameters [75], is in line with the observation of Pandyan et al. that the MAS is inadequate in characterizing the stretch reflex [40, 45]. Furthermore, Calota et al. highlighted the limitation of repetitive stretching in measurements of the DSRT and TSRT. Several studies have demonstrated an attenuation of the muscular resistance with repetitive stretching in both stroke and spinal cord injury patients [83, 84]. Further, repetitive stretching has been proven to result in elongation of muscle fascicles and an increase in sarcomere numbers [85]. Whereas time-dependent changes in motoneuronal excitability in healthy nervous systems have been reported to occur when the interval between muscle contractions is smaller than 6 seconds [86], the MSM protocol was designed with an inter-stretch interval of 10 seconds. In fact, repetitive stretching is also a problem when measuring the resistance to passive movement, whereas evidence suggests that the torque response to passive stretch decreases up to 50% after 20 to 30 cycles. This decrease has been attributed to changes in the viscoelastic properties of muscles [75]. The TSRT is believed to be influenced by both central and peripheral inputs, but the mechanical changes in motoneurons are considered to have less effect on it [78].

Although the stretch reflex seems to be the most used neurophysiological measurement method, the tendon reflex and H-reflex, which are also EMG-based, have gained momentum and established their advantage in spasticity measurement. These methods are concentrated around the same neuronal pathway but differ in the way that the reflex is elicited. As discussed, the stretch reflex is stimulated with a passive movement. However, the tendon reflex is based on a mechanical stimulus, while the H-reflex is the response to electrical stimulation.

The Hoffmann reflex or H-reflex was first described by Paul Hoffmann in 1910 and is presently used to characterize the excitability of the alpha-motoneurons. The H-reflex differs from the mechanically induced stretch reflex, whereas it bypasses the muscle spindles. It can, therefore, give valuable information on the modulation of the monosynaptic reflex activity in the spinal cord in spastic patients. The H-reflex, which is either a compound action potential or a group of essentially concurrent action potentials from neighboring muscle fibers, is elicited using a short duration and low-intensity electrical stimulus to excite sensory Ia afferent fibers. When the intensity of the stimulus is increased, motor axons are activated and send action potentials directly to the neuromuscular junction. This evokes another EMG response, which is termed the M-wave [87]. Either the H-reflex latency or the Hmax/Mmax ratio, which is the ratio of the maximum amplitudes (in V) of the waves and is generally considered an index of peripheral reflex excitability [88], are used to quantify the H-reflex [44]. Additionally, the Hslp/Mslp ratio was developed to evaluate the motoneuron excitability while eliminating the effect of changes in the peripheral region of the monosynaptic reflex arc [89]. The H-reflex parameters have been confirmed to be sensitive to the presence of spasticity and an increase in the Hmax/Mmax ratio and a decrease in the H-reflex latency have been shown to be correlated with increases in spasticity [11, 88, 90]. However, a lot of factors, including muscle activity, sensory input, state of consciousness, and age, produce a large variability in the measurement of the H-reflex [91], and the Hmax/Mmax ratio has been shown to have a large intersubject variability [92]. Furthermore, several studies on the H-reflex have demonstrated no or poor correlation to clinical scales [44, 90, 93, 94].

The F-wave is also frequently analyzed in neurophysiological examination of spasticity. The Fwave is evoked due to backfiring of the alpha motor neurons in the anterior horn of the spinal cord. When a distal nerve is simulated an antidromic impulse travels to the spinal cord, where a few of the motor neurons backfire. This backfiring generates an orthodromic impulse that elicits a small muscle contraction [95]. In order to prevent a contamination of the F-wave with the overlapping of the H-reflex, a supramaximal stimulation of the nerve is performed whereas the H-reflex is only evoked with low-intensity stimulations [96]. Abnormalities in the latency and amplitude of the Fwave have been suggested to be more sensitive to spasticity than the H-reflex [97].

Pauri et al. [98] performed transcranial magnetic stimulation, generating muscle evoked potentials (MEP) to evaluate the effect of botulinum toxin-A injection in spastic muscles. Additionally, they analyzed the effect of the treatment on the H-reflex and the F-wave. They reported significant changes in the MEP latency and the central conduction time but a lack of modulation of the H-reflex and F-wave characteristics. They postulated that their results could be explained by perceiving spasticity as a tonic noise maintaining the potential of descending pathway neurons and their transmission at the spinal a-motoneuron levels at a condition closer to their excitability threshold.

Jang et al. investigated the relationship between neurophysiological measures and clinical scales in children with CP after a botulinum toxin-A treatment and found that the amplitude of the tendon reflex had the strongest correlation with the MTS [93]. The tendon reflex is not only dependent on the excitability of alpha motoneurons but also involves the fusimotor system. It can, therefore, be argued that it is more sensitive to spasticity than the H-reflex [91]. The tendon reflex is initiated by tapping a tendon, generally the patellar tendon [99] or the Achilles tendon [93]. The reflex is then characterized by an output measure such as the time interval to an EMG response, bounce-back forces, or joint torque response [100]. Consequently, measurements of the tendon reflex are not always EMG-based. In particular, Zhang et al. [101] found that parameters based on the torque response correlated better with clinical scales than an EMG-based parameter. Using a tendon hammer with a force sensor mounted at its head along with a torque sensor, they measured the tendon tapping force, quadriceps EMG signals, and knee joint extension torque when initiating a tendon reflex in spastic MS patients. The impulse response of the tendon reflex was then calculated with the tendon tapping force as the system input and the reflex torque as the system output. They then derived three parameters to characterize the shape and amplitude of the tendon reflex impulse response, namely the tendon reflex gain (Gtr [cm]), the contraction rate (Rc [m/s]), and the reflex loop delay (td [ms]). Gtr was defined as the system gain, Rc as Gtr divided by the contraction time, and td as the interval from the onset of the tapping force to the onset of a torque response. In fact, those parameters were found to correlate better with clinical scales, such as the Ashworth scale, than the peak EMG reflex signal.

Electromechanical delay (EMD) is defined as the time between the onset of EMG activity to the onset of biomechanical force or movement, and therefore describes the time needed for electrochemical muscle activation, crossbridge formation, and elastic stretch [102]. Granata et al. [99] used the concept of the EMD to quantify the tendon reflex using the tendon tap as a stimulus to elicit muscle activation. They reported a decreased EMD in spastic muscle and attributed it to increased musculotendinous stiffness. In fact, EMD has been shown to be inversely proportional to stiffness [103]. Further, a reduced EMD in spastic patients suggests that the frequency of the peak response of muscles introduced to sinusoidal perturbations must be higher in spastic patients than normal subjects. This is in line with the results of Gottlieb et al. [104] who applied sinusoidal torques at different frequencies to the ankle joint and recorded the joint angle, torque, and EMG. Their results demonstrated a tendency toward higher resonance frequencies in spastic muscles than in normal muscles.

6. Onset detection

Most of the neurophysiological methods are dependent upon the onset of muscle activity, which is determined from the EMG data. The onset detection can be a challenging task, especially when the EMG response or the signal-to-noise ratio (SNR) is low. Most studies have exploited the amplitude of the EMG signal to detect the onset [105], either by visual inspection or by setting a threshold [106]. A common threshold used is two standard deviations above the mean baseline value of the EMG signal, which has been reported to be inadequate in low spasticity subjects [52]. In fact, onset detection methods based on the amplitude of the signal are sensitive to noise and their performance reduces as the SNR of the surface EMG signal is decreased [105]. Several methods have been developed to compensate for this, such as the double threshold detector, which was especially designed for gait analysis [107] and wavelet template matching [108] along with methods utilizing statistical criterion determination [109, 110]. However, these methods are computationally intense, which can be problematic in the clinical setting. The Teager-Kaiser energy operator (TKE), which computes the instantaneous energy changes of signals made up of a single frequency varying in time, was formulated to address these problems [111]. The TKE operator is nonlinear and is sensitive to the instantaneous amplitude and frequency of the signal. Since increases in both frequency and amplitude accompany the firing of a motor unit, the difference between the EMG signal and background noise becomes clearer in the Teager-Kaiser domain [112]. Consequently, onset detection methods, such as visual detection, threshold algorithms, and statistical approaches, will perform better when the TKE operator is included in the signal conditioning [111]. However, the TKE operator is primarily effective against noise with Gaussian distribution [105]. Another type of noise that can affect the signal quality is spurious background spikes. These spikes can develop due to motion artifacts at the skin-electrode surface or because of interference from a radio transmission and electrical wires. Zhang et al. [105] developed an onset detection method based on sample entropy that can highlight bursts of EMG activity but has low sensitivity to spurious spikes. Sample entropy is a measure of the complexity and randomness of a system. When muscle activity is elicited an increase in the complexity of the EMG signal follows, which is not true for spurious background spikes. Conditioning the signal with the sample entropy algorithm, therefore, facilitates muscle onset detection. At last, the use of the Hilbert-Huang transform (HHT) in onset detection will be briefly discussed. The HHT, which is applicable to nonstationary and nonlinear signals, is based on the concept of empirical mode decomposition that can break down complex signals into finite intrinsic mode functions [113]. The transform combines both nonlinear dynamics and time-frequency analysis and is therefore strongly suitable for EMG signal processing [114]. Furthermore, the HHT and entropy analysis have been combined into a method termed the Hilbert-Huang transform marginal spectrum entropy (HMSEN), which has shown effectiveness in seizure detection of electroencephalography (EEG) signals [115]. Hu et al. [114] utilized the HMSEN and the root-mean-square (RMS) of sEMG signals to develop a novel clinical assessment method for spasticity. The method identifies the stretch reflex onset from the sEMG signal using the HMSEN and then compares the RMS of the baseline of the signal to the RMS of a fixed length of signal obtained directly after the detected onset. The difference is then used to quantify spasticity.

7. Imaging techniques

Several medical imaging modalities have been used to aid in spasticity measurement. Positron emission tomography (PET) and magnetic resonance imaging (MRI) have been used to assess spasticity in stroke patients but are relatively unused in clinical practice [11]. Conventional B-mode ultrasonography has also been used to quantify spasticity by determining muscle architectural parameters, including muscle thickness, fascicle length, and pennation angle [116]. Evidence suggests that these architectural parameters have significantly lower values in spastic muscles [117, 118], although the decrease of fascicle length in children with CP has been disputed [119]. The parameters have been shown to have good reliability [120], but they do not supply information on the muscle stiffness. The muscle stiffness can, however, be quantified using elastography, which is a newly developed imaging technique. Elastography is based on applying stress to tissues and measuring the displacement [118] and has been used to measure the flexibility of muscles, tendons, and nerves, and thereby quantifying spasticity [121]. Several different elastography techniques have been introduced and are classified based on the method used to develop stress and measure the displacement. These methods include sonoelastography, shear wave elastography, transient elastography, and acoustic radiation force elastography, which are all based on ultrasound [119] along with magnetic resonance elastography [122]. Of those techniques, sonoelastography, which is based on applying compression to the target tissue by hand, is the most used [118, 123]. Sonoelastographic measurements have been proven to be able to differentiate between spastic and unaffected muscles but do not correlate with the MAS [113] or muscle architecture parameters obtained with B-mode ultrasonography [118]. Shear wave elastography is also frequently used in spasticity quantification and has been shown to be promising in monitoring the structural and viscoelastic properties of spastic muscles [124]. Shear wave elastography is based on using the ultrasound probe to generate transient shear waves in the muscle. The shear waves are then detected again with the probe as they travel along the muscle fibers, and their speed is used to quantify muscle stiffness [125]. Shear wave elastography has been shown to be feasible in measuring spasticity [126], but high sensitivity to the measurement conditions has also been reported, resulting in a low reliability [124]. Generally, the quantification of elastographic data is done visually by using color grading [118] or by calculating elastic moduli [124, 125]. Additionally, a new five-point scale called the muscle elastography multiple sclerosis score

(MEMS) has been developed to quantify the elastography results based on the elasticity and distribution of muscle fibers [121].

8. Multidimensionality

The majority of the spasticity measurement methods developed during the last decade take advantage of instrumented approaches, which has increased their reliability remarkably. However, the complexity of the spasticity phenomenon further requires that these methods incorporate multidimensional parameters. Evidence suggests that clinical scales, biomechanical, and neurophysiological parameters of spasticity measurement have poor correlation [10, 12, 19, 127], so combining these methods is beneficial to be able to distinguish every aspect of the spasticity. In a recent study, McGibbon et al. [50] integrated biomechanical and neurophysiological parameters relevant for spasticity quantification using a wearable sensor system. They proposed a kinematic model of spasticity, which the parameters were extracted from. The model is based on constructing a motion curve of elbow stretch and comparing it to a reference curve. In healthy subjects, a consistency can be found between the reference curve and the actual motion curve, which cannot be identified in spastic subjects. Using the kinematic model, they further managed to obtain the spastic muscle interference force without an external force transducer device. Kristinsdóttir et al. used results from the pendulum test and sEMG recordings to construct a spasticity quantification parameter called the reflex period [128]. Bar-On et al. [51] also combined biomechanical and neurophysiological methods, integrating several sEMG and torque-related parameters explored around the maximum velocity, and comparing them between velocity conditions in order to assess the spasticity in children with CP. They reported that their parameters were sensitive to spasticity [51] and provided a more comprehensive assessment than clinical scales [129]. Interestingly, Falisse et al. [130] utilized this assessment method along with 3D gait analysis to develop spasticity models and recognized that a model relying on feedback from muscle force, and its time derivative (dF/dt) was best suited in explaining muscle activity during passive stretches and gait. This is consistent with a recent theory suggesting that muscle spindle receptors encode information about muscle force instead of length [131].

Mirbagheri et al. [21] managed to separate the corresponding contributions of neural and muscular components to the overall joint stiffness by using the integration of multidimensional signals. They applied pseudorandom binary sequence perturbations to joints of spastic patients and used a parallel cascade system identification technique to process the signals and quantify the different components. Their results revealed no correlation between either component and the MAS score [12]. Wu et al. [43] developed a four-dimensional characterization of spasticity, which includes the joint angle, velocity, torque, and torque change rate, in order to systematically quantify catch angle and spasticity. Centen et al. [132] developed a robotic exoskeleton to identify kinematic characteristics of resistance to passive movement in spastic subjects. They extracted seven parameters that described the resistance to passive movement from their measurements and found that two of them were suited to differentiate patients from healthy subjects. These parameters were peak velocity, which was the most effective in identifying spasticity, and the between arm-peak velocity difference, which used the less affected side of the subject as a reference.

Advances in statistical methodologies, such as the development of machine learning algorithms, have been beneficial in managing the large datasets that accompany the analysis of multiple parameters. Zhang et al. used a supervised regression learning algorithm to process biomarkers and yield evaluation scores from a simple examination procedure using wearable surface EMG and inertial sensors [133]. The biomarkers were extracted from the previously mentioned kinematic [50] and lambda [76] models, which were constructed from the recorded data.

9. Discussion and conclusions

In this review, multiple aspects of spasticity measurement have been discussed. The review was focused on four essential classes of quantification methods, namely clinical scales, imaging techniques, biomechanical, and neurophysiological methods. Clinical scales, which are based on initiating a brisk dorsiflexion movement of the relaxed ankle and grading the resistance, are the most prevalent methods for clinical assessment of spasticity. The Ashworth and Tardieu scales have been most widely used but recently there has been development in the field, with new scales such as the ASAS [38] and SPAT [48] being created. Clinical scales that allow for two or more different velocities in the dorsiflexion movement have been shown to have higher reliability than those based on a single velocity [32, 39]. Clinical scales are advantageous in the sense that they are clinically feasible and do not require heavy equipment and instrumentation, but their main limitation is that they are based on a subjective assessment. Therefore, quantified comparison of the severity of spasticity of a muscle from time to time or between persons is limited.

Biomechanical methods are based on quantifying the resistance of a joint, most often by measuring force and torque using dynamometers [16]. Most often passive movement is used to elicit spasticity, but voluntary movement has also been shown to be correlated with the severity of spasticity [57]. The Wartenberg pendulum test, which was introduced in the 1950s, can be classified as a biomechanical measurement method, whereas it is based on the oscillatory resistance characteristics of the lower limbs [58]. The instrumentation of the pendulum test, for example, with sEMG, goniometers [64], and magnetic tracking systems [63], has made its results more reliable and turned it into a promising method to use in clinical settings. The quantification of the angle of catch, which is included in the MTS protocol [69], can also be perceived as a biomechanical measurement method.

Neurophysiological methods are based on quantifying muscle activity, and thereby predicting neural mechanisms. A big share of neurophysiological methods is based on quantifying the stretch reflex and its threshold of elicitation, which is usually defined using velocity or angular coordinates [52, 78]. Quantification of the H-reflex and tendon reflex are two other prevalent methods that belong to the neurophysiological class. In fact, these methods are all quantifying the same physical phenomenon, the stretch reflex, but differ in the way that the reflex is evoked. The stretch reflex, which is a monosynaptic spinal pathway, can be activated using passive movement, a mechanical stimulus, or electrical stimulation and measurement methods that make use of the stretch reflex can be classified accordingly. The H reflex and the F-wave are based on electrical stimulation, the tendon reflex is based on a mechanical stimulus (a tendon tap), and the stretch reflex is based on passive movement. Neurophysiological methods can be further classified into methods that are based on EMG recordings and those who are not. When EMG signals are brought into play the question of how to detect the muscle onset arises. Visual detection is frequently used but methods based on the amplitude of the signal are sensitive to noise. Consequently, methods based on energy and sample entropy have demonstrated better results [105, 114].

Imaging techniques have also been used quantify spasticity. Conventional B-mode ultrasonography can determine architectural parameters of muscles, such as muscle thickness, fascicle length, and pennation angle, which have been shown to have lower values in spastic patients [116]. Elastography, which is based on applying stress to tissues and measuring the displacement, has also been used for spasticity quantification. Elastography is advantageous, whereas it can measure muscle stiffness, which has been shown to be a good indicator of spasticity [126].

Spasticity quantification methods can further be classified according to whether they are instrumented or not. A subclassification of instrumented approaches is based on whether the limb is moved by another individual or a mechatronic device during the measurement. The instrumentation of quantification methods generally improves their accuracy [53]. At last, measurement methods can be categorized based on the dimensionality of the signals obtained. Unidimensional methods are limited when it comes to measuring spasticity, whereas its complexity requires a combination of physiological parameters for accurate classification. It has been shown that methods from the four different classes mentioned have poor correlation internally, which emphasizes the use of multidimensional parameters [2, 10, 19, 127].

To conclude, this review has provided a general overview of the methods used to quantify spasticity hitherto. No conclusion was made on the most desirable method to measure spasticity, although the benefits of instrumentation and multidimensionality are emphasized. However, the review can hopefully aid in distinguishing which methods are the most promising and eventually pave the ground for establishing a gold standard for spasticity measurement.

In order to be able to accurately quantify spasticity, there has to be a consensus on its definition and fundamental mechanisms. According to Lance's definition [6], spasticity is a hyperexcitability of the stretch reflex. However, few of the methods are directly measuring this core of the pathology but rather its consequences. In particular, if the gamma motor neuron system can be directly stimulated, a better understanding of the sensitivity of the reflex mechanisms can be obtained. Also, a deeper understanding of the interplay between the muscle spindles and the spinal neural network could pave the way for a better quantification method. Ultimately, as spasticity research progresses, its quantification methods will improve. In the meantime, this review of current methodologies and knowledge will hopefully be of value for future research.

Abbreviations

SCI	spinal cord injury
CP	cerebral palsy
MS	multiple sclerosis
AS	Ashworth scale
MAS	modified Ashworth scale
TS	Tardieu scale
MTS	modified Tardieu scale
ASAS	the Australian Spasticity assessment scale
SPAT	the Spasticity test

RTPM	resistance to passive movement
PROM	passive range of motion
SPAT	spasticity test
RMS	root-mean-square
EMG	electromyography
sEMG	surface electromyography
AOC	angle of catch
SR	stretch reflex
DSRT	dynamic stretch reflex threshold
TSRT	tonic stretch reflex threshold
MEP	muscle evoked potentials
EMD	electromechanical delay
SNR	signal-to-noise ratio
TKE	Teager-Kaiser energy operator
HHT	Hilbert-Huang transform
HMSEN	Hilbert-Huang transform marginal spectrum entropy
EEG	electroencephalography
PET	Positron emission tomography
MRI	magnetic resonance imaging
EGM	electrogram

Author details

Kristjana Ósk Kristinsdóttir[1,2], Samuel Ruipérez-Campillo[2,3,4,5] and Þórður Helgason[1*]

1 Health Technology Center, Reykjavik University – Landspitali-University Hospital, Reykjavik, Iceland

2 Department of Bioengineering, University of California, Berkeley, USA

3 School of Medicine, Stanford University, Palo Alto, USA

4 Department of Computer Science, ETH Zürich, Zürich, Switzerland

5 ITACA Institute, Universitat Politecnica de Valencia, Spain

*Address all correspondence to: thordur@landspitali.is

References

[1] Kuo C-L, Hu G-C. Post-stroke spasticity: A review of epidemiology, pathophysiology, and treatments. International Journal of Gerontology. 2018;**12**(4):280-284

[2] Elbasiouny SM, Moroz D, Bakr MM, Mushahwar VK. Management of spasticity after spinal cord injury: Current techniques and future directions. Neurorehabilitation and Neural Repair. 2010;**24**(1):23-33

[3] Shamsoddini A, Amirsalari S, Hollisaz M-T, Rahimnia A, Khatibi-Aghda A. Management of spasticity in children with cerebral palsy. Iranian Journal of Pediatrics. 2014;**24**(4):345

[4] Barnes M, Kent R, Semlyen J, McMullen K. Spasticity in multiple sclerosis. Neurorehabilitation and Neural Repair. 2003;**17**(1):66-70

[5] Li S, Francisco GE. New insights into the pathophysiology of post-stroke spasticity. Frontiers in Human Neuroscience. 2015;**9**:192

[6] Lance JW. Symposium Synopsis, in Spasticity: Disordered Motor Control. In: Feldman RG, Young RR, Koella WP, editors. Chicago: Yearbook Medical; 1980. pp. 485-494

[7] Young RR. Spasticity: A review. Neurology. 1994;**44**(11 Suppl 9): S12-S20

[8] Pandyan A, Gregoric M, Barnes M, et al. Spasticity: Clinical perceptions, neurological realities and meaningful measurement. Disability and Rehabilitation. 2005;**27**(1–2):2-6

[9] Sanger TD, Delgado TD, Gaebler-Spira D, Hallett M, Mink JW, T. F. on Childhood Motor Disorders, et al. Classification and definition of disorders causing hypertonia in childhood. Pediatrics. 2003;**111**(1):e89-e97

[10] Malhotra S, Cousins E, Ward A, et al. An investigation into the agreement between clinical, biomechanical and neurophysiological measures of spasticity. Clinical Rehabilitation. 2008;**22**(12):1105-1115

[11] Thibaut A, Chatelle C, Ziegler E, Bruno M-A, Laureys S, Gosseries O. Spasticity after stroke: Physiology, assessment and treatment. Brain Injury. 2013;**27**(10):1093-1105

[12] Alibiglou L, Rymer WZ, Harvey RL, Mirbagheri MM. The relation between ashworth scores and neuromechanical measurements of spasticity following stroke. Journal of Neuroengineering and Rehabilitation. 2008;**5**(1):1-14

[13] Burke D, Wissel J, Donnan GA. Pathophysiology of spasticity in stroke. Neurology. 2013;**80**(3 Supplement 2): S20-S26

[14] Trompetto C, Marinelli L, Mori L et al. Pathophysiology of spasticity: Implications for neurorehabilitation. BioMed Research International. 2014: 354906

[15] Bhimani R, Anderson L. Clinical understanding of spasticity: Implications for practice. Rehabilitation Research and Practice. 2014:279175

[16] van den Noort JC, Scholtes VA, Harlaar J. Evaluation of clinical spasticity assessment in cerebral palsy using inertial sensors. Gait & Posture. 2009; **30**(2):138-143

[17] Carr L. Development and reorganization of descending motor

pathways in children with hemiplegic cerebral palsy. Acta Paediatrica. 1996;**85**: 53-57

[18] Jobin A, Levin MF. Regulation of stretch reflex threshold in elbow flexors in children with cerebral palsy: A new measure of spasticity. Developmental Medicine and Child Neurology. 2000; **42**(8):531-540

[19] Willerslev-Olsen M, Lorentzen J, Sinkjær T, Nielsen JB. Passive muscle properties are altered in children with cerebral palsy before the age of 3 years and are difficult to distinguish clinically from spasticity. Developmental Medicine & Child Neurology. 2013; **55**(7):617-623

[20] Lindberg PG, Gäverth J, Islam M, Fagergren A, Borg J, Forssberg H. Validation of a new biomechanical model to measure muscle tone in spastic muscles. Neurorehabilitation and Neural Repair. 2011;**25**(7):617-625

[21] Mirbagheri M, Barbeau H, Ladouceur M, Kearney R. Intrinsic and reflex stiffness in normal and spastic, spinal cord injured subjects. Experimental Brain Research. 2001; **141**(4):446-459

[22] Gäverth J, Sandgren M, Lindberg PG, Forssberg H, Eliasson A-C. Test-retest and inter-rater reliability of a method to measure wrist and finger spasticity. Journal of Rehabilitation Medicine. 2013;**45**(7):630-636

[23] Booth CM, Cortina-Borja MJ, Theologis TN. Collagen accumulation in muscles of children with cerebral palsy and correlation with severity of spasticity. Developmental Medicine and Child Neurology. 2001;**43**(5):314-320

[24] Romanini L, Villani C, Meloni C, Calvisi V. Histological and morphological aspects of muscle in infantile cerebral palsy. Italian Journal of Orthopaedics and Traumatology. 1989; **15**(1):87-93

[25] Lieber RL, Steinman S, Barash IA, Chambers H. Structural and functional changes in spastic skeletal muscle. Muscle & Nerve: Official Journal of the American Association of Electrodiagnostic Medicine. 2004;**29**(5): 615-627

[26] Stecco A, Stecco C, Raghavan P. Peripheral mechanisms contributing to spasticity and implications for treatment. Current Physical Medicine and Rehabilitation Reports. 2014;**2**(2): 121-127

[27] Lieber RL, Runesson E, Einarsson F, Fridén J. Inferior mechanical properties of spastic muscle bundles due to hypertrophic but compromised extracellular matrix material. Muscle & Nerve: Official Journal of the American Association of Electrodiagnostic Medicine. 2003;**28**(4):464-471

[28] Desloovere K, Bar-On L. Challenges of instrumented spasticity assessment. Developmental medicine & Child neurology. 2013;**55**(7):586-587

[29] Sköld C. Spasticity in spinal cord injury: Self- and clinically rated intrinsic fluctuations and intervention-induced changes. Archives of Physical Medicine and Rehabilitation. 2000;**81**(2):144-149

[30] Bajd T, Vodovnik L. Pendulum testing of spasticity. Journal of Biomedical Engineering. 1984;**6**(1):9-16

[31] Tyson S, Connell L. How to measure balance in clinical practice. A systematic review of the psychometrics and clinical utility of measures of balance activity for neurological

conditions. Clinical Rehabilitation. 2009; **23**(9):824-840

[32] Boyd RN, Graham HK. Objective measurement of clinical findings in the use of botulinum toxin type a for the management of children with cerebral palsy. European Journal of Neurology. 1999;**6**:s23-s35

[33] Ashworth B. Preliminary trial of carisoprodol in multiple sclerosis. Practitioner. 1964;**192**:540-542

[34] Charalambous CP. Interrater reliability of a modified ashworth scale of muscle spasticity. In: Classic Papers in Orthopaedics. Springer; 2014. pp. 415-417

[35] Ansari NN, Naghdi S, Moammeri H, Jalaie S. Ashworth scales are unreliable for the assessment of muscle spasticity. Physiotherapy Theory and Practice. 2006;**22**(3):119-125

[36] Patrick E, Ada L. The tardieu scale differentiates contracture from spasticity whereas the ashworth scale is confounded by it. Clinical Rehabilitation. 2006;**20**(2):173-182

[37] Paulis WD, Horemans HL, Brouwer BS, Stam HJ. Excellent test–retest and inter-rater reliability for Tardieu scale measurements with inertial sensors in elbow flexors of stroke patients. Gait & Posture. 2011;**33**(2):185-189

[38] Love S, Gibson N, Smith N, Bear N, Blair E, A. C. P. R. Group. Interobserver reliability of the Australian spasticity assessment scale (asas). Developmental Medicine and Child Neurology. 2016;**58**: 18-24

[39] Mehrholz J, Wagner K, Meissner D, et al. Reliability of the modified Tardieu scale and the modified ashworth scale in adult patients with severe brain injury: A comparison study. Clinical Rehabilitation. 2005;**19**(7):751-759

[40] Pandyan AD, Price CI, Barnes MP, Johnson GR. A biomechanical investigation into the validity of the modified ashworth scale as a measure of elbow spasticity. Clinical Rehabilitation. 2003;**17**(3):290-294

[41] Cooper A, Musa IM, Van Deursen R, Wiles CM. Electromyography characterization of stretch responses in hemiparetic stroke patients and their relationship with the modified ashworth scale. Clinical Rehabilitation. 2005;**19**(7): 760-766

[42] Condliffe EG, Clark DJ, Patten C. Reliability of elbow stretch reflex assessment in chronic post-stroke hemiparesis. Clinical Neurophysiology. 2005;**116**(8):1870-1878

[43] Wu Y-N, Park H-S, Chen J-J, Ren Y, Roth EJ, Zhang L-Q. Position as well as velocity dependence of spasticity—Four-dimensional characterizations of catch angle. Frontiers in Neurology. 2018;**9**: 863

[44] Pisano F, Miscio G, Del Conte C, Pianca D, Candeloro E, Colombo R. Quantitative measures of spasticity in post-stroke patients. Clinical Neurophysiology. 2000;**111**(6):1015-1022

[45] Pandyan AD, Johnson GR, Price CI, Curless RH, Barnes MP, Rodgers H. A review of the properties and limitations of the ashworth and modified ashworth scales as measures of spasticity. Clinical Rehabilitation. 1999;**13**(5):373-383

[46] Olver J, Esquenazi A, Fung V, Singer B, Ward A. Botulinum toxin assessment, intervention and aftercare for lower limb disorders of movement and muscle tone in adults: International

consensus statement. European Journal of Neurology. 2010;**17**:57-73

[47] Sheean G, Lannin N, Turner-Stokes L, Rawicki B, Snow B. Botulinum toxin assessment, intervention and after-care for upper limb hypertonicity in adults: International consensus statement. European Journal of Neurology. 2010;**17**: 74-93

[48] Scholtes V, Dallmeijer A, Becher J. The spasticity test: A clinical instrument to measure spasticity in children with cerebral palsy, Eff multilevel botulinum toxin type A Compr Rehabil Child with Cereb palsy. 2007. pp. 29–64

[49] Banky M, Clark RA, Mentiplay BF, Olver JH, Kahn MB, Williams G. Toward accurate clinical spasticity assessment: Validation of movement speed and joint angle assessments using smartphones and camera tracking. Archives of Physical Medicine and Rehabilitation. 2019;**100**(8):1482-1491

[50] McGibbon CA, Sexton A, Jones M, O'Connell C. Elbow spasticity during passive stretch-reflex: Clinical evaluation using a wearable sensor system. Journal of Neuroengineering and Rehabilitation. 2013;**10**(1):1-14

[51] Bar-On L, Aertbeliën E, Wambacq H, et al. A clinical measurement to quantify spasticity in children with cerebral palsy by integration of multidimensional signals. Gait & Posture. 2013;**38**(1): 141-147

[52] Calota A, Feldman AG, Levin MF. Spasticity measurement based on tonic stretch reflex threshold in stroke using a portable device. Clinical Neurophysiology. 2008;**119**(10):2329-2337

[53] Sloot LH, Bar-On L, van der Krogt MM, et al. Motorized versus manual instrumented spasticity assessment in children with cerebral palsy. Developmental Medicine and Child Neurology. 2017;**59**(2):145-151

[54] Banky M, Ryan HK, Clark R, Olver J, Williams G. Do clinical tests of spasticity accurately reflect muscle function during walking: A systematic review. Brain Injury. 2017; **31**(4):440-455

[55] Pandyan A, Price C, Rodgers H, Barnes M, Johnson G. Biomechanical examination of a commonly used measure of spasticity. Clinical Biomechanics. 2001;**16**(10):859-865

[56] Kumar RT, Pandyan AD, Sharma AK. Biomechanical measurement of post-stroke spasticity. Age and Ageing. 2006; **35**(4):371-375

[57] Wang H, Huang P, Li X, Samuel OW, Xiang Y, Li G. Spasticity assessment based on the maximum isometrics voluntary contraction of upper limb muscles in post-stroke hemiplegia. Frontiers in Neurology. 2019;**10**:465

[58] Wartenberg R. Pendulousness of the legs as a diagnostic test. Neurology. 1951; **1**(1):18-18

[59] Fowler EG, Nwigwe AI, Ho TW. Sensitivity of the pendulum test for assessing spasticity in persons with cerebral palsy. Developmental Medicine and Child Neurology. 2000;**42**(3): 182-189

[60] Syczewska M, Lebiedowska MK, Pandyan AD. Quantifying repeatability of the wartenberg pendulum test parameters in children with spasticity. Journal of Neuroscience Methods. 2009; **178**(2):340-344

[61] Whelan A, Sexton A, Jones M, O'Connell C, McGibbon CA. Predictive value of the pendulum test for assessing knee extensor spasticity. Journal of Neuroengineering and Rehabilitation. 2018;**15**(1):1-12

[62] White H, Uhl TL, Augsburger S, Tylkowski C. Reliability of the three-dimensional pendulum test for able-bodied children and children diagnosed with cerebral palsy. Gait & Posture. 2007;**26**(1):97-105

[63] Bohannon RW, Harrison S, Kinsella-Shaw J. Reliability and validity of pendulum test measures of spasticity obtained with the polhemus tracking system from patients with chronic stroke. Journal of Neuroengineering and Rehabilitation. 2009;**6**(1):1-7

[64] Yeh CH, Young HWV, Wang CY, et al. Quantifying spasticity with limited swinging cycles using pendulum test based on phase amplitude coupling. IEEE Transactions on Neural Systems and Rehabilitation Engineering. 2016;**24**(10): 1081-1088

[65] Leonard CT, Stephens JU, Stroppel SL. Assessing the spastic condition of individuals with upper motoneuron involvement: Validity of the myotonometer. Archives of Physical Medicine and Rehabilitation. 2001; **82**(10):1416-1420

[66] Li X, Shin H, Li S, Zhou P. Assessing muscle spasticity with myotonometric and passive stretch measurements: Validity of the myotonometer. Scientific Reports. 2017;7(1):1-7

[67] Leonard CT, Brown JS, Price TR, Queen SA, Mikhailenok EL. Comparison of surface electromyography and myotonometric measurements during voluntary isometric contractions. Journal of Electromyography and Kinesiology. 2004;**14**(6):709-714

[68] Aarrestad DD, Williams MD, Fehrer SC, Mikhailenok E, Leonard CT. Intra-and interrater reliabilities of the myotonometer when assessing the spastic condition of children with cerebral palsy. Journal of Child Neurology. 2004;**19**(11):894-901

[69] Tardieu G. A la recherche d'une technique de mesure de la spasticite. Revista de Neurologia. 1954;**91**:143-144

[70] Wu Y-N, Ren Y, Goldsmith A, Gaebler D, Liu SQ, Zhang L-Q. Characterization of spasticity in cerebral palsy: Dependence of catch angle on velocity. Developmental Medicine and Child Neurology. 2010;**52**(6): 563-569

[71] Lynn B-O, Erwin A, Guy M, et al. Comprehensive quantification of the spastic catch in children with cerebral palsy. Research in Developmental Disabilities. 2013;**34**(1):386-396

[72] Thilmann A, Fellows S, Garms E. The mechanism of spastic muscle hypertonus: Variation in reflex gain over the time course of spasticity. Brain. 1991; **114**(1):233-244

[73] Lee WA, Boughton A, Rymer WZ. Absence of stretch reflex gain enhancement in voluntarily activated spastic muscle. Experimental Neurology. 1987;**98**(2):317-335

[74] Powers R, Marder-Meyer J, Rymer W. Quantitative relations between hypertonia and stretch reflex threshold in spastic hemiparesis. Annals of Neurology: Official Journal of the American Neurological Association and the Child Neurology Society. 1988;**23**(2): 115-124

[75] Sorinola IO, White CM, Rushton DN, Newham DJ. Electromyographic response to manual

passive stretch of the hemiplegic wrist: Accuracy, reliability, and correlation with clinical spasticity assessment and function. Neurorehabilitation and Neural Repair. 2009;**23**(3):287-294

[76] Feldman AG. Once more on the equilibrium-point hypothesis (λ model) for motor control. Journal of Motor Behavior. 1986;**18**(1):17-54

[77] O'Sullivan M, Eyre J, Miller S. Radiation of phasic stretch reflex in biceps brachii to muscles of the arm in man and its restriction during development. The Journal of Physiology. 1991;**439**(1):529-543

[78] Levin MF, Feldman AG. The role of stretch reflex threshold regulation in normal and impaired motor control. Brain Research. 1994;**657**(1–2):23-30

[79] Mullick AA, Musampa NK, Feldman AG, Levin MF. Stretch reflex spatial threshold measure discriminates between spasticity and rigidity. Clinical Neurophysiology. 2013;**124**(4):740-751

[80] Levin MF, Selles RW, Verheul MH, Meijer OG. Deficits in the coordination of agonist and antagonist muscles in stroke patients: Implications for normal motor control. Brain Research. 2000; **853**(2):352-369

[81] Musampa NK, Mathieu PA, Levin MF. Relationship between stretch reflex thresholds and voluntary arm muscle activation in patients with spasticity. Experimental Brain Research. 2007;**181**(4):579-593

[82] Pisano F, Miscio G, Colombo R, Pinelli P. Quantitative evaluation of normal muscle tone. Journal of the Neurological Sciences. 1996;**135**(2):168-172

[83] Hornby TG, Kahn JH, Wu M, Schmit BD. Temporal facilitation of spastic stretch reflexes following human spinal cord injury. The Journal of Physiology. 2006;**571**(3):593-604

[84] Nuyens GE, De Weerdt WJ, Spaepen AJ Jr, Kiekens C, Feys HM. Reduction of spastic hypertonia during repeated passive knee movements in stroke patients. Archives of Physical Medicine and Rehabilitation. 2002;**83**(7):930-935

[85] Gao F, Ren Y, Roth EJ, Harvey R, Zhang L-Q. Effects of repeated ankle stretching on calf muscle–tendon and ankle biomechanical properties in stroke survivors. Clinical biomechanics. 2011; **26**(5):516-522

[86] Gorassini M, Yang JF, Siu M, Bennett DJ. Intrinsic activation of human motoneurons: Reduction of motor unit recruitment thresholds by repeated contractions. Journal of Neurophysiology. 2002;**87**(4):1859-1866

[87] Palmieri RM, Ingersoll CD, Hoffman MA. The Hoffmann reflex: Methodologic considerations and applications for use in sports medicine and athletic training research. Journal of Athletic Training. 2004;**39**(3):268

[88] Tekgül H, Polat M, Tosun A, Serdaroğlu G, Gökben S. Electrophysiologic assessment of spasticity in children using h-reflex. The Turkish Journal of Pediatrics. 2013;**55**(5): 519-523

[89] Higashi T, Funase K, Kusano K, et al. Motoneuron pool excitability of hemiplegic patients: Assessing recovery stages by using h-reflex and m response. Archives of Physical Medicine and Rehabilitation. 2001;**82**(11):1604-1610

[90] Bakheit A, Maynard V, Curnow J, Hudson N, Kodapala S. The relation between ashworth scale scores and the excitability of the α motor neurones in

patients with post-stroke muscle spasticity. Journal of Neurology, Neurosurgery & Psychiatry. 2003;**74**(5):646-648

[91] Voerman GE, Gregorič M, Hermens HJ. Neurophysiological methods for the assessment of spasticity: The Hoffmann reflex, the tendon reflex, and the stretch reflex. Disability and Rehabilitation. 2005;**27**(1–2):33-68

[92] Levin MF, Hui-Chan C. Are h and stretch reflexes in hemiparesis reproducible and correlated with spasticity? Journal of Neurology. 1993; **240**(2):63-71

[93] Jang D-H, Sung IY, Kang YJ. Usefulness of the tendon reflex for assessing spasticity after botulinum toxin-a injection in children with cerebral palsy. Journal of Child Neurology. 2013;**28**(1):21-26

[94] Naghdi S, Ansari NN, Abolhasani H, Mansouri K, Ghotbi N, Hasson S. Electrophysiological evaluation of the modified tardieu scale (mts) in assessing poststroke wrist flexor spasticity. Neuro Rehabilitation. 2014;**34**(1):177-184

[95] Fisher MA. F-waves–physiology and clinical uses. The Scientific World-Journal. 2007;**7**:144-160

[96] Panayiotopoulos C, Chroni E. F-waves in clinical neurophysiology: A review, methodological issues and overall value in peripheral neuropathies. Electroencephalography and Clinical Neurophysiology/Electromyography and Motor Control. 1996;**101**(5): 365-374

[97] Joodaki M, Olyaei G, Bagheri H. The effects of electrical nerve stimulation of the lower extremity on h-reflex and f-wave parameters. Electromyography and Clinical Neurophysiology. 2001;**41**(1): 23-28

[98] Pauri F, Boffa L, Cassetta E, Pasqualetti P, Rossini PM. Botulinum toxin type-a treatment in spastic paraparesis: A neurophysiological study. Journal of the Neurological Sciences. 2000;**181**(1–2):89-97

[99] Granata KP, Ikeda AJ, Abel MF. Electromechanical delay and reflex response in spastic cerebral palsy. Archives of Physical Medicine and Rehabilitation. 2000;**81**(7):888-894

[100] Zhang L-Q, Xu D, Liao W, Rymer WZ. A quantitative and convenient method of evaluating tendon reflex and spasticity. In: Proceedings of the First Joint BMES/EMBS Conference. 1999 IEEE Engineering in Medicine and Biology 21st Annual Conference and the 1999 Annual Fall Meeting of the Biomedical Engineering Society. Cat. N. Vol. 1. Atlanta, GA, USA: IEEE; 1999. p. 549

[101] Zhang L-Q, Wang G, Nishida T, Xu D, Sliwa JA, Rymer WZ. Hyperactive tendon reflexes in spastic multiple sclerosis: Measures and mechanisms of action. Archives of Physical Medicine and Rehabilitation. 2000;**81**(7):901-909

[102] Norman RW, Komi PV. Electromechanical delay in skeletal muscle under normal movement conditions. Acta Physiologica Scandinavica. 1979;**106**(3):241-248

[103] Corcos DM, Gottlieb GL, Latash ML, Almeida GL, Agarwal GC. Electromechanical delay: An experimental artifact. Journal of Electromyography and Kinesiology. 1992;**2**(2):59-68

[104] Gottlieb GL, Agarwal GC, Penn R. Sinusoidal oscillation of the ankle as a means of evaluating the spastic patient. Journal of Neurology, Neurosurgery & Psychiatry. 1978;**41**(1): 32-39

[105] Zhang X, Zhou P. Sample entropy analysis of surface EMG for improved muscle activity onset detection against spurious background spikes. Journal of Electromyography and Kinesiology. 2012;**22**(6):901-907

[106] Hodges PW, Bui BH. A comparison of computer-based methods for the determination of onset of muscle contraction using electromyography. Electroencephalography and Clinical Neurophysiology/Electromyography and Motor Control. 1996;**101**(6): 511-519

[107] Bonato P, D'Alessio T, Knaflitz M. A statistical method for the measurement of muscle activation intervals from surface myoelectric signal during gait. IEEE Transactions on Biomedical Engineering. 1998;**45**(3): 287-299

[108] Merlo A, Farina D, Merletti R. A fast and reliable technique for muscle activity detection from surface EMG signals. IEEE Transactions on Biomedical Engineering. 2003;**50**(3): 316-323

[109] Micera S, Sabatini AM, Dario P. An algorithm for detecting the onset of muscle contraction by EMG signal processing. Medical Engineering & Physics. 1998;**20**(3):211-215

[110] Staude GH. Precise onset detection of human motor responses using a whitening filter and the log-likelihood-ratio test. IEEE Transactions on Biomedical Engineering. 2001;**48**(11): 1292-1305

[111] Solnik S, Rider P, Steinweg K, DeVita P, Hortobágyi T. Teager-Kaiser energy operator signal conditioning improves EMG onset detection. European Journal of Applied Physiology. 2010;**110**(3):489-498

[112] Li X, Zhou P, Aruin AS. Teager-Kaiser energy operation of surface EMG improves muscle activity onset detection. Annals of Biomedical Engineering. 2007;**35**(9):1532-1538

[113] Huang NE, Shen Z, Long SR, et al. The empirical mode decomposition and the Hilbert spectrum for nonlinear and non-stationary time series analysis. Proceedings of the Royal Society of London. Series A: Mathematical, Physical and Engineering Sciences. 1998; **454**(1971):903-995

[114] Hu B, Zhang X, Mu J, Wu M, Wang Y. Spasticity assessment based on the Hilbert–Huang transform marginal spectrum entropy and the root mean square of surface electromyography signals: A preliminary study. Biomedical Engineering Online. 2018;**17**(1):1-20

[115] Fu K, Qu J, Chai Y, Zou T. Hilbert marginal spectrum analysis for automatic seizure detection in EEG signals. Biomedical Signal Processing and Control. 2015;**18**:179-185

[116] Yang Y-B, Zhang J, Leng Z-P, Chen X, Song W-Q. Evaluation of spasticity after stroke by using ultrasound to measure the muscle architecture parameters: A clinical study. International Journal of Clinical and Experimental Medicine. 2014;**7**(9):2712

[117] Gao F, Grant TH, Roth EJ, Zhang L-Q. Changes in passive mechanical properties of the gastrocnemius muscle at the muscle fascicle and joint levels in stroke survivors. Archives of Physical Medicine and Rehabilitation. 2009; **90**(5):819-826

[118] Kesikburun S, Yaşar E, Adıgüzel E, Güzelküçük Ü, Alaca R, Tan AK. Assessment of spasticity with sonoelastography following stroke: A feasibility study. PM&R. 2015;**7**(12): 1254-1260

[119] Drakonaki E, Allen G, Wilson D. Ultrasound elastography for musculoskeletal applications. The British Journal of Radiology. 2012;**85**(1019): 1435-1445

[120] Shortland AP, Harris CA, Gough M, Robinson RO. Architecture of the medial gastrocnemius in children with spastic diplegia. Developmental Medicine and Child Neurology. 2002;**44**(3):158-163

[121] Illomei G, Spinicci G, Locci E, Marrosu M. Muscle elastography: A new imaging technique for multiple sclerosis spasticity measurement. Neurological Sciences. 2017;**38**(3):433-439

[122] Debernard L, Robert L, Charleux F, Bensamoun SF. Analysis of thigh muscle stiffness from childhood to adulthood using magnetic resonance elastography (MRE) technique. Clinical Biomechanics. 2011;**26**(8):836-840

[123] Hong MJ, Park JB, Lee YJ, et al. Quantitative evaluation of post-stroke spasticity using neurophysiological and radiological tools: A pilot study. Annals of Rehabilitation Medicine. 2018;**42**(3):384

[124] Mathevon L, Michel F, Aubry S, et al. Two-dimensional and shear wave elastography ultrasound: A reliable method to analyse spastic muscles? Muscle & Nerve. 2018;**57**(2):222-228

[125] Brandenburg JE, Eby SF, Song P, et al. Quantifying passive muscle stiffness in children with and without cerebral palsy using ultrasound shear wave elastography. Developmental Medicine & Child Neurology. 2016; **58**(12):1288-1294

[126] Eby SF, Zhao H, Song P, et al. Quantifying spasticity in individual muscles using shear wave elastography. Radiology Case Reports. 2017;**12**(2): 348-352

[127] Biering-Sørensen F, Nielsen J, Klinge K. Spasticity-assessment: A review. Spinal Cord. 2006;**44**(12):708-722

[128] Kristinsdottir K, Magnusdottir G, Chenery B, et al. Comparison of spasticity in spinal cord injury and stroke patients using reflex period in pendulum test. European Journal of Translational Myology. 2020;**30**(1):8907

[129] Bar-On L, Van Campenhout A, Desloovere K, et al. Is an instrumented spasticity assessment an improvement over clinical spasticity scales in assessing and predicting the response to integrated botulinum toxin type a treatment in children with cerebral palsy? Archives of Physical Medicine and Rehabilitation. 2014;**95**(3):515-523

[130] Falisse A, Bar-On L, Desloovere K, Jonkers I, De Groote F. A spasticity model based on feedback from muscle force explains muscle activity during passive stretches and gait in children with cerebral palsy. PLoS One. 2018; **13**(12):e0208811

[131] Blum KP, Lamotte D'Incamps B, Zytnicki D, Ting LH. Force encoding in muscle spindles during stretch of passive muscle. PLoS Computational Biology. 2017;**13**(9):e1005767

[132] Centen A, Lowrey CR, Scott SH, Yeh T-T, Mochizuki G. Kaps (kinematic assessment of passive stretch): A tool to assess elbow flexor and extensor spasticity after stroke using a robotic exoskeleton. Journal of Neuroengineering and Rehabilitation. 2017;**14**(1):1-13

[133] Zhang X, Tang X, Zhu X, Gao X, Chen X, Chen X. A regression-based framework for quantitative assessment of muscle spasticity using combined EMG and inertial data from wearable sensors. Frontiers in Neuroscience. 2019;**13**:398